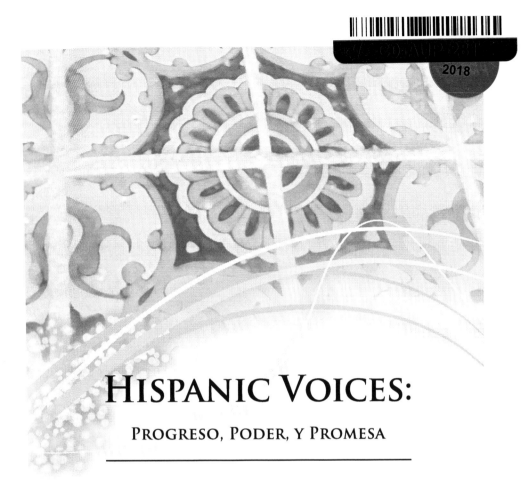

# HISPANIC VOICES:

## PROGRESO, PODER, Y PROMESA

Antonia M. Villarruel, Editor
and
Sara Torres, Co-Editor

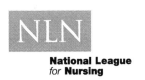

**National League**
*for* **Nursing**

National League for Nursing
61 Broadway
New York, NY 10006
212-363-5555 or 800-669-1656
www.nln.org


ISBN: 978-1-934758-16-8

Antonia M. Villarruel, PhD, RN, FAAN
University of Michigan – School of Nursing
avillar@umich.edu
Direct: (734) 615-9696


Sara Torres, PhD, RN, FAAN,
Walden University – School of Nursing
sara.torres@waldenu.edu
Direct: (651) 895-2622

Cover Design by Brian Vigorita
Art Director, Laerdal Medical Corporation



Printed in the United States of America
9 8 7 6 5 4 3 2

# HISPANIC VOICES:

## PROGRESO, PODER, Y PROMESA

# TABLE OF CONTENTS

List of Tables ................................................................................................... VII

List of Figures ................................................................................................. VIII

List of Boxes .................................................................................................. VIII

Foreword
Antonio R. Flores, PhD ....................................................................................... IX

Preface
Antonia Villarruel, PhD, RN, FAAN & Sara Torres, PhD, RN, FAAN ..................... XI

Acknowledgments ............................................................................................ XV

**Part One: Overview**

Chapter 1: The Future of the Hispanic Registered Nurse Workforce:
Improving Quality of Care and Patient Outcomes
*Robert J. Lucero, PhD, RN & Lusine Poghosyan, PhD, RN* ........................ 1

Chapter 2: The Future of Nursing for Hispanics: A Call for Transformation
in Nursing Education and Leadership
*Rosa M. Gonzalez-Guarda, PhD, MPH, RN, CPH &
Antonia M. Villarruel, PhD, RN, FAAN* ................................................... 23

**Part Two: Strategies for Recruitment and Retention of Hispanics in Nursing**

Chapter 3: Finding and Keeping Diversity in Your Program: Hispanics in the Health
Professions
*Mary Lou Bond, PhD, RN, CNE, ANEF, FAAN, Carolyn L. Cason, PhD, RN,
Pat Gleason-Wynn, PhD, RN, LCSW, Jennifer Gray, PhD, RN, Jean Ashwill,
MSN, RN, Claudia S. Coggin, PhD, CHES, Michael D. Moon, MSN, RN, CNS-CC,
CEN, FAEN, Elizabeth Trevino Dawson, DrPH, MPH, Michael Lopez, BA,
Linda Denke, PhD, RN & Susan Baxley, PhD, RN* ...................................... 41

Chapter 4: Retaining Hispanic Students in BSN Programs
*Maithe Enriquez, PhD, RN, ANP-BC & Eve McGee, MSW* ....................... 55

Chapter 5: Contributing Factors and Strategies to Address the Shortage of Hispanic
Nursing Faculty
*Evelyn Ruiz Calvillo, DNSc, RN* ............................................................. 73

Chapter 6: Juntos Podemos (Together We Can): Student-Led Mentoring -
A Key Ingredient to Increasing the Hispanic Workforce in Nursing
*Norma Martínez Rogers, PhD, RN, FAAN, Adelita G. Cantu, PhD, RN,
Theresa Villarreal, MSN, RN, ACNS-BC & Stephanie Acosta* ................... 89

**Part Three: Education Innovations**

Chapter 7:   Doctoral Studies in Nursing in Mexico: The Impact of Globalization
*Bertha Cecilia Salazar-González, PhD, RN, MA, BSN,*
*Raquel Alicia Benavides-Torres, PhD, MCE, BSN &*
*Esther C. Gallegos, PhD, RN, MBA, BSN* ...............................................99

Chapter 8:   Reflection: A Student's Perspective on Studying in Latin America
*Carmen Alvarez, PhD, RN, NP-C, CNM* ................................................113

Chapter 9:   The Use of Innovative Technologies as a Strategy to Ensure Hispanic
Nursing Student Success
*Laura Gonzalez, PhD, RN, APRN, CNE &*
*Jean Giddens, PhD, RN, FAAN* ........................................................123

Appendix A:  Author Profiles .............................................................137

Appendix B:  Instructional Self-Assessment.........................................151

Appendix C:  Program Self-Assessment ...............................................161

## List of Tables

Table 1-1    Hispanic Population 1970-2000 and Projected Hispanic Population 2020-2050 in the U.S. (Numbers in millions) .........................................5

Table 1-2    Annual Estimates of the Resident Population by Race and Hispanic Origin for the United States: July 1, 2009 ...............................................5

Table 1-3    Hispanic Origin Type Distribution of the Hispanic Population: 2007-2010 (Numbers in thousands of civilian non-institutionalized population) ..........6

Table 1-4    Regional Distribution of the Hispanic Population by Hispanic Origin Type: 2010 and 2007 (Numbers in thousands of civilian non-institutionalized population)...............................................................7

Table 1-5    Health Insurance Status by Race and Hispanic Origin Type: 2010 (Numbers in thousands of civilian non-institutionalized population) ..........8

Table 1-6    Race and Hispanic Origin of Registered Nurses in the United States: 2008.............................................................................8

Table 1-7    Regional Distribution of Registered Nurses by Race and Hispanic Origin Type in the United States: 2008 .............................................................9

Table 1-8    Years of School Completed by People 25 Years and Over by Race and Hispanic Origin: 2010 (Numbers in thousands of civilian non-institutionalized population)...........................................................11

Table 1-9    Educational Attainment of the U.S. Population 25 Years and Over by Hispanic Origin Type: 2010 and 2007 (Numbers in thousands of civilian non-institutionalized population)...........................................................12

Table 1-10    Initial Nursing Education of Employed Registered Nurses by Race and Ethnic Origin in the United States: 2008 .........................................13

Table 1-11    Highest Education of Registered Nurses by Race and Hispanic Origin in Nursing in the United States: 2008.....................................................15

Table 1-12    Students Enrolled in Entry Level Bachelor's, Master's, Doctoral (Research-Focused) Programs in Nursing, by Race and Hispanic Origin in the United States: 2010, 2005, 2001 ...............................................16

Table 2-1    Major Recommendations for the Future of Nursing (Institute of Medicine, 2011) ..............................................................25

Table 2-2    Recommended Strategies for Advancing the Future of Nursing for Hispanics ...............................................................................32

Table 4-1    Retention Strategies Targeting Underrepresented BSN Students 2002-2007 ....................................................................................61

**List of Figures**

Figure 3-1    Adapted Model of Institutional Support for Hispanic Student Degree.......44

**List of Boxes**

Box 2-1    Reflections of a Hispanic Nurse Committee Member on the IOM
            Report on the Future of Nursing (2011) ...............................................34

Box 6-1    Juntos Podemos – Reflections of a Student............................................94

Box 6-2    Juntos Podemos – Reflections of an Alumnus........................................95

It is difficult to imagine a more timely volume than *Hispanic Voices: Progreso, Poder, y Promesa*, which explores the nexus of three of the great issues of the moment: health care, education, and the emergence of Hispanics in all dimensions of American life. The 2010 census highlighted the dramatic growth of Hispanics in the United States. At 50.5 million, over 16 percent of the population, Hispanics are now the nation's largest, youngest, and fastest-growing minority (Ennis, Ríos-Vargas, & Albert, 2011). According to the Pew Hispanic Center, the Department of Labor projects that Hispanics will account for 74 percent of the growth of the labor force between 2010 and 2020 (Kochhar, 2012). The nation's need for nurses cannot be filled without even more intentional efforts to recruit and train Hispanics.

Moreover, Hispanics suffer from persisting disparities in susceptibility to various illnesses, as well as in access to adequate health care. More and better educated Hispanic nurses are a key to bringing a cultural understanding and an experiential passion to addressing these disparities. To the degree that Spanish is the first language of a substantial number of American Hispanics, a critical mass of Spanish-speaking nurses is essential to their adequate and accurate treatment.

The same poverty that incubates health disparities and health care disparities engenders disparities in educational opportunity and achievement for many Hispanics. Students from low-income families are far more likely to attend less well-funded schools, be taught by less experienced and out-of-field teachers, and have less access to academic counseling. Economic and family obligations can make post-secondary education virtually unimaginable. As a consequence, Latinos drop out of high school at three times the rate of white non-Hispanics and attend college at a far lower rate than white non-Hispanics.

These educational realities pose serious challenges for Hispanic nursing education, as well as the entire educational process. Early outreach, family and community involvement, aggressive and supportive counseling, and mentorship are not only components of a successful undergraduate recruitment strategy, but need to be continuing and guiding principles of the entire educational process.

This volume, edited by Drs. Antonia M. Villaruel and Sara Torres, constitutes an important contribution to this crucial set of issues. It brings to bear the considered and varied experience of a range of experts to address the progress, the power, and the promise of Hispanic voices in nursing.

Antonio R. Flores, PhD
President and CEO
The Hispanic Association of Colleges and Universities (HACU)

## REFERENCES

Ennis, S. R., Ríos-Vargas, M., & Albert, N. G. (2011, May). *The Hispanic population 2010: 2010 census briefs.* Retrieved from U.S. Census Bureau website: http://www.census.gov/prod/cen2010/briefs/c2010br-04.pdf

Kochhar, R. (2012, March 21). *The demographics of the jobs recovery: Employment gains by race, ethnicity, gender and nativity.* Retrieved from Pew Hispanic Center website: http://www.pewhispanic.org/2012/03/21/the-demographics-of-the-jobs-recovery/

This book is one of three in the second series by the National League for Nursing dedicated to exploring issues related to the health care and education of minorities in the United States. The first series was published in 1996 and included a book titled Hispanic Voices: Hispanic American Health Educators Speak Out. This first edition encompassed nursing education in addition to health and health care issues related to Hispanics.

For the second edition we have chosen the title Hispanic Voices: Progreso, Poder, y Promesa, or Progress, Power, and Promise. The second edition focuses on nursing education — the recruitment, retention, graduation, and leadership development of Hispanics. The themes of progress, power, and promise are prominent throughout each chapter, as are descriptions of culture-specific and effective approaches for recruitment, education, and leadership of Hispanics in nursing. The Institute of Medicine's (IOM) The Future of Nursing: Leading Change, Advancing Health (2011) report provides an important context and framework for the book. Strategies to increase and support Hispanics in nursing are aligned with committee recommendations.

## The Voices

As you read this book, you will hear the voices of Hispanic and other nurses as they share their successes and challenges related to the education of Hispanic nurses in the United States. Clearly, there has been much progress in developing effective approaches to address the lack of Hispanic representation in nursing since the first edition was published.

The development and conceptualization of this book involved many decisions regarding the selection of content and contributions from distinguished authors. Nurses with various experiences and from all levels of education and educational programs were invited to contribute. The result is a medley of powerful voices — nurses who are students, educators, clinicians, researchers, and administrators — sharing experiences and perspectives in addressing issues confronted by Hispanics in the nursing workforce. You will hear voices from Hispanic nurses with baccalaureate, master's, and doctoral degrees. You will also hear voices of Hispanic nurses who teach in all levels of higher education — associate, baccalaureate, and graduate. You will hear voices from Hispanic nurses who teach at small private colleges and at large, nationally prominent public and private universities in the U.S. and Mexico, as well as voices from small state universities. We are pleased, also, to include the voices of some students and recent graduates. We look forward with promise to their continued contributions.

We asked each author to discuss the issues he or she deemed most relevant in the education of Hispanic nurses today, rather than commission chapters on specific outcomes. The authors' freedom to explore and reveal these issues resulted in pertinent discussions of some of the major challenges and successes facing educators who work with Hispanics.

Despite a multitude of challenges, there are commonalities in the individual and institutional strategies developed to assure success in recruitment, graduation, and leadership development of Hispanic nurses. Institutional commitment to diversity and to Hispanics, dedicated faculty, supportive institutional and family environments, and learning strategies that showcase the strengths of Hispanic students are common threads in all the chapters.

## Organization and Content Overview

This book contains nine chapters organized in three distinct parts. This organization reflects major recommendations of the IOM's report The Future of Nursing: Leading Change, Advancing Health (2011) and highlights the progress, power, and promise in the education of Hispanics. Part One contains two chapters that provide an overview on past, present, and future perspectives of Hispanics in nursing, an important foundation for the remaining chapters. In Chapter 1, Lucero and Poghosyan document our progress through a historical, demographic, education, and health lens to frame contemporary issues and opportunities related to recruitment, education, and advancement of Hispanic nurses. In Chapter 2, Gonzalez-Guarda and Villarruel review the major recommendations of the IOM's report on the future of nursing and discuss the implications for Hispanic nurses related to education and leadership. In addition, Gonzalez-Guarda, a young Hispanic nurse leader and member of the IOM Committee on the Future of Nursing, reflects on and provides voice to her experience.

Part Two contains three chapters that focus on the recruitment of Hispanic students into nursing. Chapter 3, led by Bond, is a collaborative effort among 11 authors in five universities to study the perceptions of Hispanic students enrolled in health professions programs using two self-assessment inventories described at the end of the chapter and included in the appendices. The authors offer these assessment inventories as helpful in gauging and evaluating the progress in recruitment and graduation initiatives. In Chapter 4, Enriquez and McGee describe the Student Success Program, a promising comprehensive retention program for Hispanic students in a BSN program. In addition, informal retention strategies for Hispanic students are presented. Important strategies that emerged include mentoring, reaching out to parents, supplemental instruction and academic prep, social work case management, and coping with financial stress. The authors emphasize that early assessment and intervention is critical to the retention of Hispanic students. In Chapter 5, Calvillo discusses five strategies for the successful recruitment and retention of Hispanic nurses into faculty positions. Calvillo emphasizes that institutional commitment is the single most important and powerful concept in planning and developing recruitment strategies and operationalizing a successful model or plan. Rogers, Cantu, Villarreal, and Acosta describe in Chapter 6 the development and implementation of a mentorship program, Juntos Podemos, which has demonstrated success in an approach to retain

Hispanic students in a school of nursing. This comprehensive mentoring program positions students to recognize their power in meeting their own goals while they support others in their success. Additionally, we hear the voices of participants in the program who share and reflect on their own progress.

Part Three consists of three chapters that focus on innovations in education. In Chapter 7, Salazar, Benavides, and Gallegos discuss the progress of nursing education in Mexico through the development of the first PhD program in the country. The development of this program has many parallels with efforts to improve nursing education in the U.S. and highlights the benefits and opportunities in international collaboration. Alvarez, in Chapter 8, reflects on two powerful international experiences during her undergraduate career and how these experiences impacted the trajectory of her research career in nursing, as well as global opportunities for collaboration in nursing. In Chapter 9, Gonzalez and Giddens discuss two innovative learning technologies used in nursing education — virtual communities and simulation. They show how these technologies facilitate student success among Hispanic nurses.

We are proud of the stellar contributions presented in this book. These 9 chapters and additional reflections communicate a vision for Hispanics in nursing as well as a legacy of commitment, dedication, resolve, and ingenuity in addressing the complex issue of educating Hispanic nurses. We commend all the authors for their contributions, which are just a small reflection of their work in educating Hispanic nurses. This book is an important step in building evidence-based strategies to increase the number of Hispanics in nursing. Although this book provides only a glimpse into the issues regarding the education of Hispanics in nursing, the progress, power, and promise realized to date provide hope that we will reach the ultimate goal of equity and justice within our profession and for the people in our communities.

*Antonia M. Villarruel, PhD, RN, FAAN*
*Editor*
*Professor and Nola J. Pender Collegiate Chair*
*School of Nursing*
*University of Michigan*

*Sara Torres, PhD, RN, FAAN*
*Co-Editor*
*Associate Dean and Professor*
*School of Nursing*
*Walden University*

# ACKNOWLEDGMENTS

This second edition, *Hispanic Voices: Progreso, Poder, y Promesa*, reflects the dedication and commitment of a cadre of people. While it is difficult to acknowledge by name the many individuals whose support, encouragement, and dedicated work made this book a reality, I would like to express my thanks to the many people who assisted in the writing and publication of the second edition of this book. First, gracias to the National League for Nursing Press for initiating this series of books devoted to the education and health of diverse ethnic/racial groups in the United States. Their enthusiastic support of this project is commendable. We deeply appreciate the support of Janice Brewington, NLN consultant for NLN publications, and Justine Fitzgerald, project manager for NLN publications, who read and reviewed this document to insure a high standard of excellence. Their patience, input, interest, and guidance are appreciated. Thanks also to our copy editor Melissa Gillis and to our book designer Brian Vigorita. And a special thanks to Manuela Sifuentes who came to work with us at an opportune time. She was our right hand at a crucial time in the development of this book. I am especially thankful for the contributions and support of co-editor Dr. Sara Torres. She led the way in editing the first edition of Hispanic Voices and has been unselfish in her support and work on this second edition. Finally, we are grateful for the contributions of all the authors, not only for their respective chapters, but for their dedication to educating the next generation of Hispanic nurses. Through their work they have demonstrated what this book exemplifies — poder, progreso, y promesa!

Antonia M. Villarruel, PhD, RN, FAAN
Editor
Hispanic Voices
Summer 2012

# CHAPTER 1

## THE FUTURE OF THE HISPANIC REGISTERED NURSE WORKFORCE: IMPROVING QUALITY OF CARE AND PATIENT OUTCOMES

*Robert J. Lucero, PhD, RN*
*Lusine Poghosyan, PhD, RN*

The future of nursing is now! The demand for managing chronic conditions, primary care, prevention and wellness, and the prevention of adverse events, as well as the provision of mental health services, school health services, long-term care, and palliative care is increasing. Congress and the president of the United States signed into federal law, in 2010, comprehensive health legislation known as the Affordable Care Act (ACA). The ACA represents the broadest reforms to the U.S. health care system since the 1965 creation of the Medicare and Medicaid programs. With the enactment of this law, an estimated 32 million previously uninsured Americans will gain access to insurance coverage by 2014. In the near term, the new health care laws will result in great challenges and exciting opportunities related to improvements in delivering safe, high-quality, effective health care services.

The profession of nursing represents the largest sector of health professions, with more than three million registered nurses (RNs) in the United States. Registered nurses bring a steadfast commitment to patient care, improved safety and quality, and better outcomes. However, how well the RN population reflects the general population may be inextricably tied to quality improvement and patient outcomes. The Institute of Medicine's (IOM) report (2011) The Future of Nursing: Leading Change, Advancing Health has called on the nursing profession to "increase the diversity of students to create a workforce prepared to meet the demands of diverse populations across the lifespan" (p. S-12). Thus for the nursing profession, health care reform provides an opportunity to meet the demand for safe, high-quality, patient-centered, and equitable health care services with greater emphasis placed on increasing the diversity of the RN workforce. The current and next generations of Hispanic RNs have key roles to play as primary care providers, educators, leaders, and scientists for a more comprehensive, patient-centered health care system.

This chapter explores historical, contextual, and contemporary issues that are important to consider as nurse-leaders, stakeholders, and policymakers advocate for increasing the diversity of the future nurse workforce and ultimately, improving the quality of care and patient outcomes

## A BRIEF EDUCATION HISTORY OF HISPANICS IN THE UNITED STATES

In this brief account, we will highlight pivotal events that continue to influence the educational attainment of Hispanics in the U.S. and implications for creating a pool of potential nursing students and nurses. The history of Hispanics can be understood by examining subgroups (e.g., Mexicans, Puerto Ricans, Cubans, South or Central Americans) that populate different U. S. geographical regions (e.g., Northeast, Midwest, South, and West). However, this brief history focuses on the largest subgroups, including Mexican Americans, Puerto Ricans, and Cubans, while acknowledging the growing migration of Hispanics from Central and South America to the U.S.

## Mexican Americans

The Mexican American War of 1846 and the Treaty of Guadalupe Hidalgo granted Mexican nationals a "right of passage" living in the territory conquered by the U.S. The Treaty lead to the following two important consequences: (a) the annexation of a sizeable portion of Mexico now known as Arizona, California, Colorado, Nevada, New Mexico, and Texas, and (b) the decision by many Mexicans to stay in the "U.S." and become U.S. citizens, a condition of the Treaty. These events set the stage for the marginalization of Mexican Americans (Valencia, 1998). These new Americans became a prime target for economic exploitation with the construction of railroads. Moreover, this domination extended to educational opportunities because schooling was placed under the control of U.S. governmental agencies at the local, territorial, state, and/or federal levels (MacDonald, 2001). The transition from Mexican nationals to American citizens was void of any efforts on the part of the U.S. government to assimilate these "foreigners" (Rodriquez, 1992). The result was a large Spanish-speaking population that was linguistically and culturally isolated in their newfound country.

The critical education needs of Mexicans in the U.S. would not surface until after World War II. The GI Bill (1944) gave thousands of Mexican-American veterans an opportunity to attend college. This educational benefit unintentionally exposed a little known Pandora's box. Public schools had not been designed to provide equal educational opportunities to bilingual, bi-cultural Hispanics in the U.S. (Rodriquez, 1992). The largest proportion of the U.S. Spanish-speaking population in the 1960s with the greatest concentration of elementary and secondary level school age students was of Mexican descent. During this period, there were growing Hispanic civil rights movements. Chicano (i.e., a subgroup of Mexicans) leaders and students pushed for the implementation of bilingual and bi-cultural training for teachers, elimination of tracking based on standardized testing, improvement and replacement of inferior school facilities, removal of racist teachers and administrators, and inclusion of Mexican history and culture into the curriculum (Gutierrez, 1996).

The de-industrialization and emerging globalization of the late twentieth century have indirectly influenced the education of Mexican Americans. The loss of manufacturing jobs and industries eroded the tax base of urban communities making it difficult for municipalities to maintain public schools. These were the same schools Mexican Americans relied on to prepare them for higher education opportunities, including professional nursing.

## Puerto Ricans

The educational experience of the Puerto Rican population in the U.S. can be characterized by three important historical events. The first event was the colonization of Puerto Rico. As a colony of the U.S., the focus was on teaching Puerto Rican children the English language. This focus was reinforced by mandates from the U.S. government (Alvarez-Gonzalez, 1999).

The second event was and continues to be the back and forth travel of Puerto Ricans from the U.S. to Puerto Rico. This has had a negative impact on the consistency of Puerto Rican children's education (Nieto, 1998). The third event emerged around the time when Mexican Americans were pursuing equal education rights. The Puerto Rican community began organizing to address the worsening educational experiences of Puerto Rican children and social problems. Like the Mexican-American movement, two issues were confronted — the need for bilingual education and greater participation of Puerto Rican educators.

### Cubans

For Cubans, the educational experience has been starkly different from Mexicans and Puerto Ricans. The majority of Cuban immigrants or political refugees were from the middle or upper classes of Cuban society. Cubans' status as political refugees of communism and the Cuban Revolution during the 1950s provided them easier access to educational opportunities. The U.S. federal government worked closely with local communities to set up English language programs. For example, in Dade County, Florida, the U.S. federal government helped establish the Cuban Refugee Program through annual agreements with the county school system (Sullivan & Pedraza-Bailey, 1979).

Many of the issues that adversely influenced the educational experience of Hispanics in the past continue to plague the schools most Hispanic children attend in the U.S. and influence their abilities to pursue post-secondary education. Researchers have found that Hispanic students entering kindergarten are more likely to be rated lower than white students by their teachers, regardless of their academic ability (Reardon & Galindo, 2003). Moreover, Hispanics are most likely to be enrolled in large public schools with large class sizes, and these schools are also more likely to be underfunded and deficient in resources (ERIC, 2004).

## WHO ARE U.S. HISPANICS

Hispanics account for one of every seven persons in the U.S. The growth rate of the U.S. Hispanic population in the last part of the twentieth century led to a nearly four-fold increase from 1970 to 2000 (see Table 1.1). The U.S. Census Bureau has projected that this growth rate is unlikely to slow during the first half of the twenty-first century. The Hispanic population increased by an estimated 12.5 million persons from 2000-2010. By 2050, Hispanics are likely to account for nearly one of every four persons, or 25 percent of the population. The continued growth of the Hispanic population will add to the challenges and opportunities faced by the nursing profession to address issues of social justice (e.g., access to care), health equity (e.g., equal treatment), and equal opportunity (e.g., recruitment and retention of the next generation of Hispanic nurses).

*Table 1-1*

Hispanic Population 1970-2000 and Projected Hispanic Population 2020-2050 in the U.S.
(Numbers in millions)

| | Census | | | | Projections[1] | | | | |
|---|---|---|---|---|---|---|---|---|---|
| | 1970 | 1980 | 1990 | 2000 | 2010 | 2020 | 2030 | 2040 | 2050 |
| n | 9.6 | 14.6 | 22.4 | 35.3 | 47.8 | 59.7 | 73.0 | 87.7 | 102.6 |
| percent | 4.7 | 6.4 | 9.0 | 12.5 | 15.5 | 17.8 | 20.1 | 22.3 | 24.4 |

Source: U.S. Census Bureau, 2006. 1970, 1980, 1990, and 2000 Decennial Censuses.
[1]Population Projections July 1, 2010 to July 1, 2050.

The Hispanic population reflects perhaps the most diverse group of individuals in the U.S. While 92 percent of Hispanics report they are descendants of the white race, their family backgrounds also include black, American Indian or Alaskan Native, Asian, Native Hawaiian or Pacific Islander, and mixed races (see Table 1.2). The diversity of Hispanics will continue to evolve as they marry with individuals from other racial and ethnic backgrounds. In 2010, according to the Pew Research Center, 26 percent of newlywed Hispanics married someone who was not Hispanic (Taylor et al., 2012). Because the majority of Americans accept intermarriage, this upward trend among all racial and ethnic groups is unlikely to change in the short-term, increasing the diversity of Hispanics (Taylor et al. ).

*Table 1-2*

Annual Estimates of the Resident Population by Race and Hispanic Origin for the United States: July 1, 2009

| Year | Race | Not Hispanic | Hispanic[1] |
|---|---|---|---|
| 2009 | White | 199,851,240 | 44,447,153 |
| | Black | 37,681,544 | 1,959,516 |
| | AIAN | 2,360,807 | 790,477 |
| | Asian | 13,686,083 | 327,871 |
| | NHPI | 448,510 | 129,843 |
| | ≥ 2 Races | 4,559,042 | 764,464 |
| | TOTAL | 258,587,226 | 48,419,324 |

Source: U.S. Census Bureau, 2010a. 1Hispanic origin is considered an ethnicity, not a race. Hispanics may be of any race. Abbreviations: Black = Black or African American; AIAN = American Indian and Alaska Native; NHPI = Native Hawaiian and other Pacific Islander. The original race data from Census 2000 are modified to eliminate the "Some Other Race" category.

The overall growth of the U.S. Hispanic population from 2007-2010 was impacted greatly by increases in the Mexican, Puerto Rican, and Cuban populations (see Table 1.3). During this period, the Puerto Rican population grew by 14 percent, while the Mexican and Cuban populations grew by 10 percent each. In contrast, all other Hispanic persons (who are aggregated by the census) increased only by four percent. The future growth of the Hispanic population will be driven by births in the United States, rather than immigration from abroad (Taylor et al., 2012). Although the U.S. Hispanic population is now relatively youthful compared with the general population, they will account for a growing proportion of the middle-aged and elderly in the future.

*Table 1-3*

Hispanic Origin Type Distribution of the Hispanic Population: 2007-2010 (Numbers in thousands of civilian non-institutionalized population[1])

**Hispanic Origin type[2]**

| Year | Total Hispanic | Mexican | Puerto Rican | Cuban | Other[3] |
|------|----------------|---------|--------------|-------|----------|
| 2010 | 48,901 | 32,071 | 4,406 | 1,826 | 10,598 |
| 2009 | 47,485 | 31,550 | 4,224 | 1,647 | 10,063 |
| 2008 | 46,026 | 30,272 | 4,030 | 1,612 | 10,112 |
| 2007 | 44,854 | 29,145 | 3,868 | 1,661 | 10,180 |

Source: U. S. Census Bureau, 2012. *Hispanic population of the United States.* [1]This includes armed forces living off post or with their families on post. [2]Hispanic refers to people whose origin is Mexican, Puerto Rican, Cuban, Spanish-speaking Central or South American countries, or other Hispanic/Latino, regardless of race. Central American totals exclude Mexican. [3]This category includes Dominicans and people who responded to "Hispanic," "Latino," or provided other general terms.

The Pew Hispanic Center reported that the Hispanic population more than doubled from the year 2000 to 2010 in nine U.S. states, including the Southeastern states of Alabama, Arkansas, Kentucky, Mississippi, North Carolina, Tennessee, and South Carolina, as well as Maryland and South Dakota (Passel, Cohn, & Lopez, 2011). Over time, Hispanic subgroups have settled in different geographical epicenters in the U.S. Table 1.4 shows the regional distribution of the Hispanic population in the U.S. Since 2007, there has been little change in where most Hispanics live in the U.S. Mexicans (52.0 percent), Puerto Ricans (55.5 percent), and Cubans (79.1 percent) tend to be located in the West, Northeast, and South, respectively. However, a large proportion of Mexicans (35.8 percent) and Puerto Ricans (28.8 percent) live in the South. Because the U.S. Census Bureau's definition of the South includes Texas and Florida, it is likely that "southern" Mexicans and Puerto Ricans live in these states, respectively. The smallest proportion of the Hispanic population lives in the Midwest. Hispanics from Central and South American are distributed similarly across the

Northeastern (29.4 percent), Southern (34.8 percent), and Western (31.1percent) regions of the U.S. The distribution of the Hispanic population has important health implications, including health and disease surveillance and access to primary care.

*Table 1-4*

Regional Distribution of the Hispanic Population by Hispanic Origin Type: 2010 and 2007 (Numbers in thousands of civilian non-institutionalized population)

**Hispanic Origin type[2]**

| Year | Region | Total Hispanic | | Mexican | | Puerto Rican | | Cuban | | Other[3] | |
|---|---|---|---|---|---|---|---|---|---|---|---|
| | | n | % | n | % | n | % | n | % | n | % |
| 2010 | Northeast | 6,693 | 13.7 | 944 | 2.9 | 2,445 | 55.5 | 183 | 10.0 | 3,123 | 29.4 |
| | Midwest | 3,926 | 8.0 | 2,985 | 9.3 | 403 | 9.1 | 44 | 2.4 | 495 | 4.7 |
| | South | 17,877 | 36.6 | 11,475 | 35.8 | 1,267 | 28.8 | 1,445 | 79.1 | 3,690 | 34.8 |
| | West | 20,404 | 41.7 | 16,667 | 52.0 | 291 | 6.6 | 154 | 8.4 | 3,292 | 31.1 |
| | **Total** | **48,900** | | **32,071** | | **4,406** | | **1,826** | | **10,600** | |
| 2007 | Northeast | 6,131 | 13.7 | 728 | 2.5 | 2,130 | 55.1 | 172 | 10.3 | 3,100 | |
| | Midwest | 3,900 | 8.7 | 2,923 | 10.0 | 365 | 9.4 | 45 | 2.7 | 566 | |
| | South | 15,954 | 35.6 | 10,037 | 34.4 | 1,128 | 29.2 | 1,325 | 79.8 | 3,464 | |
| | West | 18,870 | 42.1 | 15,456 | 53.0 | 245 | 6.3 | 118 | 7.1 | 3,050 | |
| | **Total** | **44,855** | | **29,144** | | **3,868** | | **1,660** | | **10,180** | |

Source: U.S. Census Bureau, 2010b, 2007. *Current Population Survey, Annual Social and Economic Supplement.* 1Regions are described by the CPS glossary of subject concepts at www.census.gov/population/www/cps/cpsdef.html

Hispanics make up the largest proportion of uninsured individuals in the U.S. (see Table 1.5). Nearly one of every three Hispanics is without health care insurance, which can negatively impact their ability to obtain timely high quality care. The uninsured are more than twice as likely as the insured to lack a health care provider (Johnson & Johnson, 2010). Although lacking health insurance raises the likelihood of not having access to care, having health insurance does not necessarily guarantee access.

At present, Hispanics have a lower prevalence of many conditions than the population as a whole. Hispanics, however, have a higher prevalence of diabetes and higher obesity rates. Since U.S.-born Hispanics tend to be less healthy than Hispanic immigrants, this compositional change may further predispose the population to chronic illness. Moreover, accessing preventative health care is difficult for a large proportion of Hispanics.

*Table 1-5*

Health Insurance Status by Race and Hispanic Origin Type: 2010 (Numbers in thousands of civilian non-institutionalized population)

| Health Insurance | | Insurance | | No Insurance | |
|---|---|---|---|---|---|
| Race and Hispanic Origin Type | Total | n | % | n | % |
| White | 243,232 | 205,938 | 84.7 | 37,385 | 15.3 |
| Black | 39,031 | 30,899 | 79.2 | 8,132 | 20.8 |
| Asian | 14,332 | 11,731 | 81.9 | 2,600 | 18.1 |
| All Hispanics | 48,901 | 33,081 | 67.6 | 15,820 | 32.4 |
| Mexican | 32,071 | 21,046 | 65.6 | 11,025 | 34.4 |
| Puerto Rican | 4,406 | 3,646 | 82.7 | 761 | 17.3 |
| Cuban | 1,826 | 1,334 | 73.0 | 492 | 27.0 |
| Other Hispanic | 10,598 | 7,056 | 66.6 | 3,542 | 33.4 |

Source: U.S. Census Bureau, 2010b. *Current Population Survey, Annual Social and Economic Supplement.*

# HISPANIC REGISTERED NURSE WORKFORCE

The rapid growth and size of the U.S. Hispanic population offers considerable reasons for the nursing profession to pay particular attention to the recruitment of Hispanic nursing students. Hispanic RNs remain underrepresented when compared with the distribution of the general U.S. population (see Table 1.6). The Hispanic RN population is only 3.6 percent of the total RN population in the U.S. Nevertheless, the population of Hispanic RNs increased two-fold from 54,861 in 2000 to 109,387 in 2008. This increase was greater than the increases for all other groups of RNs. Based on the size of the RN population in 2008, a growth rate of approximately 100 percent among Hispanic RNs would be needed every 10 years until 2040 for them to reflect the composition of the general Hispanic population.

*Table 1-6*

Race and Hispanic Origin of Registered Nurses in the United States: 2008

**Race[1] and Hispanic Origin[2]**

| Year | Total | | White | Black | AIAN | Asian | NHPI | Hispanic | > 2 Races |
|---|---|---|---|---|---|---|---|---|---|
| 2008 | 3,063,162 | n | 2,549,302 | 165,352 | 8,571 | 169,454 | 9,528 | 109,387 | 51,568 |
| | | % | 83.2 | 5.4 | 0.3 | 5.5 | 0.3 | 3.6 | 1.7 |
| 2004 | 2,909,357 | n | 2,380,529 | 122,495 | 9,453 | 84,383 | 5,594 | 44,550 | 41,244 |
| | | % | 81.8 | 4.2 | 0.3 | 2.9 | 0.2 | 1.7 | 1.4 |
| 2000 | 2,696,540 | n | 2,333,896 | 133,041 | 13,040 | 93,415 | 6,475 | 54,861 | 32,536 |
| | | % | 86.6 | 4.9 | 0.5 | 3.5 | 0.2 | 2.0 | 1.2 |

Source: U.S. Department of Health and Human Services, Health Resources and Services Administration,

2001, 2006, 2010. *National Sample Survey of Registered Nurses 2000, 2004, and 2008.* 1This includes those who only selected one race. 2This includes those who self-identified having an ethnic background that was Hispanic/Latino or not, regardless of race. Abbreviations: AIAN = American Indian or Alaskan Native; NHPI = Native Hawaiian or Pacific Islander.

The regional distribution of the Hispanic RN population does not reflect the general RN population; however, the proportion of Hispanic RNs across geographic regions does reflect the distribution of the general Hispanic population. The majority of Hispanic RNs are located in the Southern (41 percent) and Western (35 percent) regions of the U.S. (see Table 1.7). Twenty-four percent of the Hispanic RN population is divided between the Northeast (12 percent) and Midwest (12 percent). The largest proportion of Hispanic RNs is in the West (6.5 percent), followed by the South (4.1 percent), the Northeast (2.0 percent), and the Midwest (1.7 percent). This pattern may support targeting student recruitment training efforts in locations where both a larger proportion of Hispanics live and Hispanic RNs work.

### Table 1-7

Regional Distribution of Registered Nurses by Race and Hispanic Origin Type in the United States: 2008

**Region**

|  | Northeast | | Midwest | | South | | West | |
|---|---|---|---|---|---|---|---|---|
|  | $n^2$ | % | n | % | n | % | n | % |
| Total (3,063,162) | 649,805 | 18.2 | 767,361 | 25.1 | 1,062,354 | 34.7 | 583,643 | 19.1 |
| Race and Hispanic Origin | | | | | | | | |
| White | 557,818 | 85.8 | 698,083 | 91.0 | 850,917 | 80.1 | 435,345 | 74.6 |
| Black/African American | 32,411 | 5.0 | 23,115 | 3.0 | 95,369 | 9.0 | 14,328 | 2.5 |
| Asian | 37,683 | 5.8 | 19,028 | 2.5 | 40,369 | 3.8 | 70,362 | 12.1 |
| NHPI | -- | -- | -- | -- | -- | -- | 5,154 | 1.0 |
| AIAN | -- | -- | -- | -- | -- | -- | 2,433 | 0.4 |
| ≥ 2 Races | 7,336 | 1.1 | 12,013 | 1.6 | 16,320 | 1.5 | 16,310 | 2.8 |
| Hispanic | 12,796 | 2.0 | 13,073 | 1.7 | 43,392 | 4.1 | 37,981 | 6.5 |

Source: U.S. Department of Health and Human Services, Health Resources and Services Administration, 2010. *National Sample Survey of Registered Nurses 2008.* [1]Regions are based on the U.S. Census Regions and Divisions of the United States, Geography Division. [2]Estimated numbers may not equal totals, and percent may not add to 100 because of too few cases to estimate a percent. Abbreviations: -- = Too few cases to report estimated percent.

# THE EDUCATION OF U.S. HISPANICS

### Early Childhood

The enrollment of Hispanic children in quality preschool education can provide them with a solid educational foundation. The school environment supports a learning space where children are encouraged to develop cognitive and social skills needed for long-term knowledge acquisition (Nevarez & Rico, 2007). In other words, children who acquire skills at an early age are more likely to acquire more skills as they age. Historically, Hispanic families have not enrolled their children in preschool programs at high rates. In 2004, only 55 percent of eligible Hispanic children were enrolled in a preschool program, compared to 80 percent among black and white children (Tienda & Mitchell, 2006). The primary reasons for the low enrollment of Hispanic children in preschool include the following: (a) the belief by Hispanic parents that their home environment is more conducive to the well-being of children; (b) the emphasis by Hispanic families on academic skills versus educators' emphasis on child behaviors when making decisions about preschool; (c) cost; (d) lack of transportation; (e) availability of health care (i.e. immunization requirements for enrollment); and, (f) lack of knowledge about the benefits of a preschool experience (Nevarez & Rico, 2007). Nevertheless, the enrollment rates have been increasing since 2000.

Hispanic RNs can facilitate overcoming some of the barriers to preschool enrollment expressed by Hispanic families. Hispanic RNs can play a role in educating families about the long-term benefits of early childhood education, including family and child health (e.g., family cohesiveness, mental health, and nutrition) (Deming, 2009; World Bank, 2001). Hispanic RNs can partner with community-based organizations to launch community awareness programs that provide education workshops for parents and families. Hispanic RNs can be the conduit that brings together a shared understanding of the differing viewpoints of readiness and enrollment between teachers and parents.

### Educational Trends

The number of Hispanic students graduating from college has been increasing rapidly for many years among all levels of degrees from associate through doctorate (Aud, Fox, & KewalRamani, 2010). A larger proportion of Hispanics attends college than 20 years ago. In 2000, 22 percent of 18- to 24-year-old Hispanics were enrolled in colleges and universities up from 16 percent in 1980. However, in 2010, the Census Bureau reported that 37.8 percent of Hispanic adults 25 years old and older did not have a high school diploma (see Table 1.8). This proportion is more than two times that of the next highest figure, 15.8 percent. The proportion of Hispanics 25 years old and older with a college degree (18. 9 percent) is less than half (39.1 percent) of the total population. Hispanics are well behind all other racial groups beyond the bachelor's degree. Among all races, Hispanics had the smallest proportion (3.9 percent) of individuals who have completed a master's degree or higher. There is less than one Hispanic graduate for every two non-Hispanic white and black graduates and less than one Hispanic graduate for every five Asian graduates.

*Table 1-8*

Years of School Completed by People 25 Years and Over by Race and Hispanic Origin: 2010
(Numbers in thousands of civilian non-institutionalized population[1])

**Race[1] and Hispanic Origin**

| Years of School | All Races N | % | Non-Hispanic White n | % | Black n | % | Asian n | % | Hispanic (of any race) n | % |
|---|---|---|---|---|---|---|---|---|---|---|
| Elementary or High School, no diploma | 25,488 | 12.9 | 11,007 | 7.9 | 3,638 | 15.8 | 1,048 | 11.1 | 9,795 | 37.8 |
| Elementary or GED High School, or diploma | 61,618 | 31.2 | 43,802 | 31.6 | 8,074 | 35.1 | 1,928 | 20.4 | 7,814 | 30.2 |
| College, no degree | 33,010 | 16.8 | 24,203 | 17.5 | 4,557 | 19.8 | 859 | 9.1 | 3,391 | 13.1 |
| Associate degree | 17,966 | 9.1 | 13,428 | 9.7 | 2,154 | 9.4 | 675 | 7.1 | 1,709 | 6.6 |
| Bachelor degree | 37,216 | 19.4 | 29,610 | 21.4 | 2,378 | 10.4 | 3,059 | 32.3 | 2,169 | 8.4 |
| Master's degree | 15,728 | 7.6 | 11,846 | 8.6 | 1,871 | 8.2 | 1,278 | 13.5 | 733 | 2.8 |
| Professional degree | 3,038 | 1.6 | 2,444 | 1.8 | 176 | 0.8 | 284 | 3.0 | 134 | 0.5 |
| Doctorate degree | 2,744 | 1.4 | 2,141 | 1.5 | 123 | 0.5 | 334 | 3.5 | 146 | 0.6 |
| **Total[2]** | **196,808** | | **138,481** | | **22,971** | | **9,465** | | **25,891** | |

Source: U.S. Census Bureau, 2010b. *Current Population Survey, Annual Social and Economic Supplement.* [1]Excluding members of the Armed Forces living in post barracks. [2]Elementary or High School, no diploma; Elementary or High School, GED or diploma; College, no degree; Associate's degree; Bachelor's degree; Master's degree numbers and percentages are based on a sum of multiple subcategories within each category.

*Table 1-9*

Educational Attainment of the U.S. Population 25 Years and Over by Hispanic Origin Type: 2010 and 2007 (Numbers in thousands of civilian non-institutionalized population)

**Education**

| Year | Hispanic Origin Type | | Less than H.S. | H.S | Some College or A.D. | Bachelor degree | Bachelor degree or more |
|------|---------------------|---|----------------|------|----------------------|-----------------|-------------------------|
| 2010 | Total Hispanic | N | 9,795 | 7,815 | 5,100 | 2,652 | 1,013 |
|      |                | % | 37.1 | 29.6 | 19.3 | 10.1 | 3.8 |
|      | Mexican | n | 7,002 | 4,863 | 2,813 | 1,292 | 450 |
|      |         | % | 42.6 | 29.6 | 17.1 | 7.9 | 2.7 |
|      | Puerto Rican | n | 604 | 760 | 611 | 303 | 117 |
|      |              | % | 25.2 | 31.8 | 25.5 | 12.6 | 4.9 |
|      | Cuban | n | 239 | 386 | 324 | 231 | 105 |
|      |       | % | 18.6 | 30.0 | 25.2 | 18.0 | 8.2 |
|      | Other | n | 1,951 | 1,805 | 1,353 | 826 | 341 |
|      |       | % | 31.0 | 28.8 | 21.6 | 13.2 | 5.4 |
| 2007 | Total Hispanic | N | 9,741 | 6,962 | 4,722 | 2,317 | 810 |
|      |                | % | 39.7 | 28.4 | 19.2 | 9.4 | 3.3 |
|      | Mexican | n | 7,034 | 4,236 | 2,611 | 1,069 | 311 |
|      |         | % | 46.1 | 27.8 | 17.1 | 7.0 | 2.0 |
|      | Puerto Rican | n | 575 | 663 | 574 | 235 | 120 |
|      |              | % | 26.5 | 30.6 | 26.5 | 10.9 | 5.5 |
|      | Cuban | n | 230 | 362 | 234 | 232 | 76 |
|      |       | % | 20.2 | 31.9 | 20.6 | 20.5 | 6.7 |
|      | Other | n | 1,903 | 1,700 | 1,302 | 779 | 304 |
|      |       | % | 31.8 | 28.4 | 21.7 | 13.0 | 5.1 |

Source: U.S. Census Bureau, 2010b, 2007. *Current Population Survey, Annual Social and Economic Supplement.* Abbreviations: H.S. = High School; A.D. = Associate's Degree.

# EDUCATING THE NEXT GENERATION OF HISPANIC NURSES

A lack of Hispanic students in the educational pipeline naturally constrains recruitment efforts by nursing schools. Many individuals from underrepresented groups, including Hispanics, may be unwilling to pursue a career in nursing because of inadequate family support, feelings of isolation and discrimination, lack of direction from early authority figures, and economic barriers (Amaro, Abriam-Yago, & Yoder, 2006; Gardner, 2005; Jeffreys, 2007; Loftus & Duty, 2010). The lack of diversity among faculty and administrators in nursing education programs can intensify the problem of recruiting and retaining Hispanic students in schools of nursing. Schools of nursing should reach out to these RNs who live, work, and socialize in Hispanic communities as a recruitment strategy. These academic-practice-professional partnerships can be used to facilitate mentoring among Hispanic RNs and students (Wilson, Andrews, & Leners, 2006).

## The Education of Hispanic Registered Nurses

Registered nurses' education occurs typically through three educational paths — diploma, associate's degree, and baccalaureate degree. There are few diploma programs left in the U.S. Diploma programs are traditionally based in hospitals and last three years. Notably, a small proportion (5.5 percent) of Hispanic RNs has chosen diploma programs for their initial nursing education. The most common route for initial education of RNs in the U.S. is the associate's degree program (see Table 1.10). Associate's degree programs generally require two years of nursing coursework after completion of pre-requisites that include basic science. In 2008, over 50 percent of Hispanic RNs reported that the associate's degree was their point of entry into the nursing profession. Bachelor's degree programs usually span four years of full-time education. Hispanic (39.4 percent) and Asian (69.6 percent) RNs were more likely than white (32.5 percent) and black/African-American (32.1 percent) non-Hispanic nurses to have pursued a bachelor's or higher degree.

### Table 1-10
Initial Nursing Education of Employed Registered Nurses by Race and Ethnic Origin in the United States: 2008

**Nursing Education**

| Race or Hispanic Origin | Diploma percent | Associate's Degree percent | Bachelor's Degree and higher percent |
|---|---|---|---|
| White | 19.3 | 48.2 | 32.5 |
| Black/African American | 13.2 | 54.7 | 32.1 |
| Asian | 12.6 | 17.8 | 69.6 |
| Hispanic | 5.5 | 55.1 | 39.4 |

Source: U.S. Department of Health and Human Services, Health Resources and Services Administration, 2010. *National Sample Survey of Registered Nurses 2008*.

Professional nursing is a demanding and complex practice that requires knowledgeable, skilled, independent practitioners. Researchers have identified clinical implications of degree preparation suggesting that a higher proportion of bachelor's prepared nurses (BSN) are associated with improved patient outcomes (Aiken, Clarke, Cheung, Sloane, & Silber, 2003; Estabrooks, Midodzi, Cummings, Ricker, & Giovannetti, 2005; Friese, Lake, Aiken, Silber, & Sochalski, 2008; Tourangeau et al., 2007). Associate's degree programs may provide an attractive alternative to BSN programs that may require more investment of time and money before generating a return in the form of reasonably well-paying jobs.

Advancement opportunities may be more limited for associate's degree and diploma graduates compared to RNs who have obtained a bachelor's degree or higher. Many RNs obtain additional degrees that are not specifically nursing degrees but which are related to their nursing employment (U.S. Department of Health and Human Services Health Resources and Services Administration, 2010). In 2008, 32 percent of RNs with a bachelor's or higher degree reported that their initial RN education was a diploma or an ADN, demonstrating that many RNs pursue additional degrees after completion of their initial RN education (U.S. Department of Health and Human Services Health Resources and Services Administration). Black/African-American non-Hispanic RNs were more likely than white non-Hispanic RNs to have obtained both bachelor's (41.5 percent versus 39.2 percent) and graduate degrees (16.7 percent versus 14.5 percent) (see Table 1.11). In contrast, Hispanic (45.6 percent) and Asian RNs (70.0 percent) were more likely than white or black/African-American non-Hispanic RNs to pursue a bachelor's degree (see Table 1.11). These trends present an opportunity for the nursing profession to investigate the predisposing factors related to Hispanic RNs motivation to pursue advanced nursing education.

It is important to understand what motivates and/or discourages ADN RNs to pursue advanced education. Researchers conducted focus groups with 37 Hispanic BSN RNs in six cities throughout the U.S. to identify barriers and bridges to educational mobility (Villarruel, Canales, & Torres, 2001). The RNs had initially completed their associate's degree in nursing. These RNs reported limited financial resources, English as a second language, perceived discrimination, and isolation and separateness as barriers to nursing education. Additional factors included institutional barriers (e.g., unsupportive faculty, lack of advisement, and lack of flexibility) and gender roles within the Hispanic culture (e.g., care of the family as opposed to pursuit of individual goals). In contrast, barriers for some nurses were sources of strength for others, such as positive institutional support, financial assistance, and family support. These RNs also mentioned personal factors (e.g., individual aspirations and attributes) and professional aspirations (e.g., job mobility and job security) as motivating factors for success.

*Table 1-11*

Highest Education[1] of Registered Nurses by Race and Hispanic Origin in the United States: 2008

**Highest Degree**

| Race or Hispanic Origin | Bachelor's percent | Master's or doctorate percent |
|---|---|---|
| White | 39.2 | 14.5 |
| Black/African American | 41.5 | 16.7 |
| Asian | 70.0 | 10.6 |
| Hispanic | 45.6 | 11.0 |

Source: U.S. Department of Health and Human Services, Health Resources and Services Administration, 2010. *National Sample Survey of Registered Nurses 2008.* [1]Nursing and non-nursing.

The Hispanic RN population must continue to make strides in pursuing advanced nursing degrees to contribute to the IOM's recommendation of increasing the proportion of BSN RNs to 80 percent by 2020 (IOM, 2011). A more educated Hispanic RN workforce can be better equipped to meet current and future demands of patients. The care RNs provide in hospitals depends on synthesizing and analyzing data from advanced clinical technology and complex information management systems (Cornell, Riordan, & Herrin-Griffith, 2010). Care in the community is becoming more complex as well. RNs are coordinating care for patients across multiple community agencies, helping patients manage chronic illnesses to prevent acute care hospitalizations, and using a variety of technological tools to improve the quality and effectiveness of care (Forbes & While, 2009). Table 1.12 presents the enrollment of students in bachelor's, master's, and doctoral nursing degree programs by race and Hispanic origin. All groups increased the number of students enrolled across all degree programs from 2001 to 2010 except for white doctoral students. In fact, from 2005 to 2010, across all degree programs there was a drop in white student enrollment. RN leaders must be at the forefront of making online and traditional ADN-to-BSN, LPN-to-MSN, ADN-to-MSN, and BSN-to-PhD programs more visible to Hispanic RNs.

*Table 1-12*

Students Enrolled in Entry-Level Bachelor's, Master's, Doctoral (Research-Focused) Programs in Nursing, by Race and Hispanic Origin[1] in the United States: 2010, 2005, 2001

| Year | Race and Hispanic Origin | Bachelor's | | Master's | | Doctoral | |
|---|---|---|---|---|---|---|---|
| | | N | % | N | % | N | % |
| 2010 | White* | 108,426 | 73.2 | 54,981 | 73.9 | 3,077 | 76.8 |
| | Black* | 16,165 | 10.9 | 9,613 | 12.9 | 478 | 11.9 |
| | A/NH/PI* | 12,441 | 8.4 | 5,360 | 7.2 | 217 | 5.4 |
| | AIAN | 904 | 0.6 | 572 | 0.8 | 52 | 1.3 |
| | Hispanic | 10,091 | 6.8 | 3,842 | 5.2 | 183 | 4.6 |
| | **TOTAL** | **148,027** | | **74,368** | | **4,007** | |
| 2005 | White | 88,399 | 75.9 | 32546 | 78.0 | 2,585 | 81.6 |
| | Black | 13,944 | 11.7 | 4468 | 10.7 | 313 | 9.9 |
| | A/NH/PI | 6,095 | 6.4 | 2461 | 5.9 | 144 | 4.5 |
| | AIAN | 7,500 | 0.7 | 278 | 0.7 | 21 | 0.7 |
| | Hispanic | 870 | 5.2 | 1953 | 4.7 | 104 | 3.3 |
| | **TOTAL** | **116,475** | | **41,706** | | **3,167** | |
| 2001 | White | 57081 | 54.5 | 23,485 | 59.3 | 2251 | 77.0 |
| | Black | 8934 | 8.5 | 2,551 | 6.4 | 196 | 6.7 |
| | A/NH/PI | 3931 | 3.8 | 1,425 | 3.6 | 90 | 3.1 |
| | AIAN | 504 | 0.5 | 165 | 0.4 | 10 | 0.3 |
| | Hispanic | 4460 | 4.3 | 1,170 | 3.0 | 63 | 2.2 |
| | **TOTAL** | **74,910** | | **28,796** | | **2,610** | |

Source: American Association of Colleges of Nursing, 2012. [1]Hispanic origin refers to people whose origin is Mexican, Puerto Rican, Cuban, Spanish-speaking Central or South American countries, or other Hispanic/Latino, regardless of race. *Not of Hispanic origin. Abbreviations: A/NH/PI = Asian, Native Hawaiian, or Other Pacific Islander; AIAN = American Indian or Alaskan Native

# FUTURE OPPORTUNITIES AND CHALLENGES OF HISPANIC NURSES

A culturally diverse nursing workforce is essential to meeting the health care needs of the nation's populations (Betancourt, Maina, & Soni, 2005). Given the sizeable constitution of minority populations in the U.S., the nursing profession needs to strengthen their efforts to attract and retain greater numbers of minority students, especially Hispanics. Hispanic RNs are significant contributors to the provision of health care services in the U.S. and can lead the development of models of care that address the unique needs of Hispanics.

### Quality, Access, and Value

Factors that influence clinical decisions and care delivery include uncertainty, time pressures, and both conscious and unconscious bias and stereotyping about the patient. Nurses' behavior and their clinical decisions can directly contribute to disparities in health care for patients (Institute of Medicine, 2002). A greater representation of Hispanics and other underrepresented groups in nursing has the potential to mitigate the effects of unequal care by enhancing the cultural awareness of other nurses. The goal is to improve the quality of care by increasing the cultural competence of health care providers.

There is evidence that minority health care providers are significantly more likely than their white counterparts to serve in minority and medically under-served communities (Sullivan Commission on Diversity in the Healthcare Workforce, 2004). This too may be true of Hispanic RNs based on their geographical distribution in relation to the general Hispanic population. A relatively small percentage of Hispanics (approximately 26 percent) have a health care provider that shares their background. In contrast, 82 percent of white Americans have a white health care provider (Collins et al., 2002). This disparity will not be easy to resolve in the short term. However, increasing the enrollment of Hispanics in nursing schools and promoting the educational advancement of Hispanic RNs will provide more opportunities for Hispanics to choose a health care provider who shares a similar perspective.

Increasing the representation of Hispanic RNs at all levels in the U.S. should be viewed not only as a way to increase access to high-quality care for Hispanics, but also as a business strategy for nursing schools and health care organizations. Most nursing schools in the U.S. have not yet realized the value of diversity. Diversity in higher education is critical for the development of individual and organizational skills (such as the ability to understand, learn from, and work and build consensus with individuals from different backgrounds and cultures) necessary to participate and compete globally (Sullivan Commission on Diversity in the Healthcare Workforce, 2004). There also may be valuable benefits health care organizations can derive from a greater proportion of Hispanic RNs in the U.S, including improving organizational communication, maximizing human resources, improving access to services, and improving patient satisfaction. For example, researchers found that in California, children in non-English-speaking households were more likely to lack health insurance, not have a doctor contact, go to other countries for health care, and less likely to use emergency rooms (Yu, Huang, Schwalberg, & Nyman, 2006). All of these factors affect the bottom-lines of health care organizations.

**Nursing Science**

The discovery of knowledge related to the science of nursing is necessary to providing appropriate patient care, evaluating outcomes, and eliminating health disparities. Along with an adequate representation of Hispanic RNs, meeting Hispanics' growing health care needs requires growth in the science of delivering effective care and designing health systems, as well as health promotion. Hispanic nurse scientists can be a critical link in the discovery and translation of knowledge for use by Hispanic populations. The research conducted by Hispanic nurse scientists has uncovered important health implications for Hispanics in the U.S. Advances have been made, for example, in the understanding of risk and protective factors that affect the mental health of migrant families (Siantz, Coronado, & Dovydaitis, 2010); the delivery of culturally appropriate interventions to Hispanics (Peragallo, Gonzalez-Guarda, McCabe, & Cianelli, 2011); and the development and testing of interventions to reduce HIV sexual risk among Hispanic youth (Villarruel, Jemmott, & Jemmott, 2006).

## CONCLUSION

The educational status of Hispanics in the U.S. is trending in a positive direction, and more needs to be done to promote this pattern. One result will be a larger pool of students available to attract into nursing. In spite of the currently restricted pipeline, the nursing profession has made great progress in recruiting and retaining underrepresented minority nursing students over the past decade. Nurse leaders must build on what they have learned, develop innovative strategies to recruit the next generation of Hispanic nurses, and produce sustainable resources to retain highly qualified, intellectual Hispanic registered nurses. All of this is critical if nursing is to reach the IOM's (2011) recommendation of doubling the number of nurses with a doctorate by 2020, "to add to the cadre of nurse faculty and researcher, with attention to increasing diversity" (p. S-20). A sustained focus on diversity in nursing and among nurses will help ensure that patients receive culturally relevant, high-quality care.

## REFERENCES

Aiken, L. H., Clarke, S. P., Cheung, R. B., Sloane, D. M., & Silber, J. H. (2003). Educational levels of hospital nurses and surgical patient mortality. *Journal of the American Medical Association, 290*(12), 1617-1623.

Alvarez-Gonzalez, J. J. (1999). Law, language and statehood: The role of English in the great state of Puerto Rico. *Law and Inequality, 17*, 359-443.

Amaro, D. J., Abriam-Yago, K., & Yoder, M. (2006). Perceived barriers for ethnically diverse students in nursing programs. *Journal of Nursing Education, 45*(7), 247-254.

American Association of Colleges of Nursing. (2012). *Research and Data: 10 Years of Race/Ethnicity Data Available Online.* Retrieved from http://www.aacn.nche.edu/research-data/EthnicityTbl.pdf

Aud, S., Fox, M., & KewalRamani, A. (2010). *Status and trends in the education of racial and ethnic groups* (National Center for Education Statistics 2010-015). Washington, DC: U.S. Government Printing Office.

Betancourt, J. R., Maina, A. W., & Soni, S. M. (2005). The IOM report Unequal Treatment: Lessons for clinical practice. *Delaware Medical Journal, 77*(9), 339-348.

Collins, K. S., Hughes, D. L., Doty, M. M., Ives, B. L., Edwards, J. N., & Tenney, K. (2002). *Diverse communities, common concerns: Assessing health care quality for minority Americans.* New York, NY: The Commonwealth Fund.

Cornell, P., Riordan, M., & Herrin-Griffith, D. (2010). Transforming nursing workflow, part 2: The impact of technology on nurse activities. *Journal of Nursing Administration, 40*(10), 432-439.

Deming, D. (2009). Early childhood intervention and life-cycle skill development: Evidence from Head Start. *American Economic Journal: Applied Economics, 1*(3), 111-134.

ERIC. (2004). Latinos in school: Some facts and findings, 2001. *ERIC Digest Number 162.* Retrieved February 23, 2012, from www.eric.ed.gov

Estabrooks, C. A., Midodzi, W. K., Cummings, G. G., Ricker, K. L., & Giovannetti, P. (2005). The impact of hospital nursing characteristics on 30-day mortality. *Nursing Research, 54*(2), 74-84.

Forbes, A., & While, A. (2009). The nursing contribution to chronic disease management: A discussion paper. *International Journal of Nursing Studies, 46*(1), 119-130.

Friese, C. R., Lake, E. T., Aiken, L. H., Silber, J. H., & Sochalski, J. (2008). Hospital nurse practice environments and outcomes for surgical oncology patients. *Health Services Research, 43*(4), 1145-1163.

Gardner, J. (2005). Barriers influencing the success of racial and ethnic minority students in nursing programs. *Journal of Transcultural Nursing, 16*(2), 155-162.

Gutierrez, H. J. (1996). Racial politics in Los Angeles: Black and Mexican American challenges to unequal education in the 1960s. *Southern California Quarterly, 78*(1), 51-86.

Institute of Medicine. (2002). *Unequal treatment: Confronting racial and ethnic disparities in health care.* Washington, DC: The National Academies Press.

Institute of Medicine. (2011). *The Future of nursing: Leading change, advancing health.* Washington, DC: The National Academies Press.

Jeffreys, M. R. (2007). Nontraditional students' perceptions of variables influencing retention: A multisite study. *Nurse Education, 32*(4), 161-167.

Johnson, N. J., & Johnson, L. P. (Eds.). (2010). *The care of the uninsured in America.* New York, NY: Springer.

Loftus, J., & Duty, S. (2010). Educating ethnic minority students for the nursing workforce: Facilitators and barriers to success. *Journal of the National Black Nurses Association, 21*(1), 7-16.

MacDonald, V. M. (2001). Hispanic, Latino, Chicano, or "other"?: Deconstructing the relationship between historians and Hispanic-American educational history. *History of Education Quarterly, 41*(3), 365-413.

Nevarez, C., & Rico, T. (2007). *Latino education: A synthesis of recurring recommendations and solutions in P-16 education.* New York: The College Board.

Nieto, S. (1998). Fact and fiction: Stories of Puerto Ricans in U.S. schools. *Harvard Educational Review, 68*(2), 133-163.

Passel, J. S., Cohn, D., & Lopez, M. H. (2011). *Census 2010: 50 million Latinos, Hispanics account for more than half of nation's growth in past decade.* Washington, DC: Pew Hispanic Center.

Peragallo, N., Gonzalez-Guarda, R. M., McCabe, B. E., & Cianelli, R. (in press). The efficacy of an HIV risk reduction intervention for Hispanic women. *AIDS and Behavior, 16*(5), 1316-1326.

Reardon, S., & Galindo, C. (2003). *Hispanic children and the initial transition to schooling: Evidence from the Early Childhood Longitudinal Study.* Paper presented at the National Academies/National Research Council, Panel on Hispanics in the United States, Newport Beach, CA.

Rodriquez, H. (1992). Population, economic mobility and income inequality: A portrait of Latinos in the United States, 1970-1992. *Latino Studies Journal, 3*(2), 55-86.

Siantz, M. L., Coronado, N., & Dovydaitis, T. (2010). Maternal predictors of behavioral problems among Mexican migrant farmworker children. *Journal of Family Nursing, 16*(3), 322-343.

Sullivan Commission on Diversity in the Healthcare Workforce. (2004). *Missing persons: Minorities in the health professions: A report of the Sullivan Commission on Diversity in the Healthcare Workforce.* Washington, DC: Author.

Sullivan, T. A., & Pedraza-Bailey, S. (1979). *Differential success among Cuban-American and Mexican-American immigrants: The role of policy and community.* Chicago, IL: National Opinion Research Center.

Taylor, P., Wang, W., Parker, K., Passel, J. S., Patten, E., & Motel, S. (2012). *The rise of intermarriage: Rates, characteristics vary by race and gender.* Washington, DC: Pew Research Center.

Tienda, M., & Mitchell, F. (Eds.). (2006). *Multiple origins, uncertain destinies: Hispanics and the American future*. Washington, DC: National Academies Press.

Tourangeau, A. E., Doran, D. M., McGillis Hall, L., O'Brien Pallas, L., Pringle, D., Tu, J. V., & Cranley, L. A. (2007). Impact of hospital nursing care on 30-day mortality for acute medical patients. *Journal of Advanced Nursing, 57*(1), 32-44.

U.S. Department of Health and Human Services, Health Resources and Services Administration. (2010). *The registered nurse population: Findings from the 2008 National Sample Survey of Registered Nurses*. Washington, DC: U.S. Government Printing Office.

U.S. Census Bureau. (2006). *Hispanics in the United States*. Retrieved from http://www.census.gov/population/www/socdemo/hispanic/files/Internet_Hispanic_in_US_2006.pdf

U.S. Census Bureau. (2010). *Annual Estimates of the Resident Population by Sex, Race, and Hispanic Origin for the United States: April 1, 2000 to July 1, 2009* (NC-EST2009-03). Population Estimates. Retrieved from http://www.census.gov/popest/data/national/asrh/2009/index.html

U.S. Census Bureau. (2012). *Current Population Survey Annual Social and Economic Survey.* Retrieved from http://www.census.gov/hhes/www/poverty/publications/pubs-cps.html

Valencia, R. R. (1998). From the Treaty of Guadalupe Hidalgo to "Hopwood": The educational plight and struggle of Mexican Americans in the Southwest. *Harvard Educational Review, 68*(3), 353-412.

Villarruel, A. M., Canales, M., & Torres, S. (2001). Bridges and barriers: Educational mobility of Hispanic nurses. *Journal of Nursing Education, 40*(6), 245-251.

Villarruel, A. M., Jemmott, J. B., 3rd, & Jemmott, L. S. (2006). A randomized controlled trial testing an HIV prevention intervention for Latino youth. *Archives of Pediatric & Adolescent Medicine, 160*(8), 772-777.

Wilson, V. W., Andrews, M., & Leners, D. W. (2006). Mentoring as a strategy for retaining racial and ethnically diverse students in nursing programs. *Journal of Multicultural Nursing & Health, 12*(3), 17-23.

The World Bank. (2001). *Benefits of early child development programs*. Retrieved on February 21, 2012, from http://go.worldbank.org/2AHNORUYE0

Yu, S. M., Huang, Z. J., Schwalberg, R. H., & Nyman, R. M. (2006). Parental English proficiency and children's health services access. *American Journal of Public Health, 96*(8), 1449-1455. doi: 10.2105/ajph.2005.069500

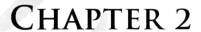

# CHAPTER 2
## THE FUTURE OF NURSING FOR HISPANICS: A CALL FOR TRANSFORMATION IN NURSING EDUCATION AND LEADERSHIP

Rosa M. Gonzalez-Guarda, PhD, MPH, RN, CPH
Antonia M. Villarruel, PhD, RN, FAAN

Increasing the number and capacity of Hispanic nurses is an imperative for improving the health of the U.S. population. Hispanics are the fastest growing minority group in the U.S. and are expected to comprise 29 percent of the general population and 23 percent of children by 2050 (Pew Research Center, 2008). Nevertheless, Hispanics are an underrepresented racial and ethnic group in the registered nurse (RN) workforce. This demographic mismatch, coupled with the increase in access to health care associated with the passage of the Patient Protection and Affordable Care Act, will result in more Hispanic consumers engaging with a health care system that is not equipped to address the unique health needs of this emergent population. The current health care delivery system requires a transformation, one that focuses on improving culturally and linguistically appropriate services, eliminating barriers to health care endured by minority groups, and creating health promotion and disease prevention programs to address health inequities affecting Hispanics and other health disparity populations. The ability to accomplish these changes will determine, to a large extent, the future health of Hispanics and the U.S. population as a whole.

Hispanic nurses represent an untapped resource in our health care delivery system that can bring about the required transformation that our health care delivery system requires to meet the needs of a diversifying U.S. population. The Institute of Medicine (IOM) has emphasized in various reports the importance of increasing the diversity of health professionals, including nurses, as a means of improving the quality and cultural appropriateness of health care services and eliminating structural causes of health disparities (IOM, 2002, 2004). However, increasing the numbers is not enough. Changes are also needed in the way that nurses, especially Hispanic nurses, are trained and deployed. In fact, the landmark IOM report, The Future of Nursing: Leading Change, Advancing Health (2011), calls for a "fundamental transformation of the nursing profession," (p. 28) one that requires us to rethink the way in which nurses are educated, deliver services and lead changes in our health care delivery system. In this chapter, we will review the major recommendations of the IOM report on the future of nursing and discuss some of the important implications that recommendations relating to education and leadership have for Hispanic nurses. We conclude with recommendations regarding what actions are necessary to ensure that there is a large and capable Hispanic nursing workforce to address the health challenges of the twenty-first century.

## THE INITIATIVE ON THE FUTURE OF NURSING

In July 2009, a major initiative on the future of nursing was established by the Robert Wood Johnson Foundation (RWJF). As a cornerstone of this initiative, an IOM Committee was tasked with examining the capacity of the nursing workforce to meet the future needs of a reformed health care delivery system and to develop action-oriented recommendations for required transformations. The committee developed eight bold recommendations (IOM, 2011, pp. 278-284) (see Table 2-1).

*Table 2-1*

Major Recommendations for the Future of Nursing (Institute of Medicine, 2011)

1. **Remove scope-of-practice barriers.** Advanced practice registered nurses should be able to practice to the full extent of their education and training.

2. **Expand opportunities for nurses to lead and diffuse collaborative improvement efforts.** Private and public funders, health care organizations, nursing education programs, and nursing associations should expand opportunities for nurses to lead and manage collaborative efforts with physicians and other members of the team to conduct research and to redesign and improve practice environments and health systems. These entities should also provide opportunities for nurses to diffuse successful practices.

3. **Implement nurse residency programs.** State boards of nursing, accrediting bodies, the federal government, and health care organizations should take actions to support nurses' completion of a transition-to-practice program (nurse residency) after they have completed a pre-licensure or advanced practice degree program or when they are transitioning into new clinical practice areas.

4. **Increase the proportion of nurses with a baccalaureate degree to 80 percent by 2020.** Academic nurse leaders across all schools of nursing should work together to increase the proportion of nurses with a baccalaureate degree from 50 to 80 percent by 2020. These leaders should partner with education accrediting bodies, private and public funders, and employers to ensure funding, monitor progress, and increase the diversity of students to create a workforce prepared to meet the demands of diverse populations across the lifespan.

5. **Double the number of nurses with a doctorate by 2020.** Schools of nursing, with support from private and public funders, academic administrators and university trustees, and accrediting bodies, should double the number of nurses with a doctorate by 2020 to add to the cadre of nurse faculty and researchers, with attention to increasing diversity.

6. **Ensure that nurses engage in lifelong learning.** Accrediting bodies, schools of nursing, health care organizations, and continuing competency educators from multiple health professions should collaborate to ensure that nurses and nursing students and faculty continue their education and engage in lifelong learning to gain the competencies needed to provide care for diverse populations across the lifespan.

7. **Prepare and enable nurses to lead change to advance health.** Nurses, nursing education programs, and nursing associations should prepare the nursing workforce to assume leadership positions across all levels, while public, private, and governmental health care decision-makers should ensure that leadership positions are available to and filled by nurses.

8. **Build an infrastructure for the collection and analysis of interprofessional health care workforce data.** The National Healthcare Workforce Commission, with oversight from the Government Accountability Office and the Health Resources and Services Administration, should lead a collaborative effort to improve research and the collection and analysis of data on health care workforce requirements. The Workforce Commission and the Health Resources and Services Administration should collaborate with state licensing boards, state nursing workforce centers, and the Department of Labor in this effort to ensure that the data are timely and publicly accessible.

From The Future of Nursing: Leading Change, Advancing Health (p. 9-15), *by Institute of Medicine, 2011, Washington, DC: National Academy of Sciences. Copyright 2011 by the National Academies of Science. Reprinted with permission from the National Academies Press.*

Great strides in implementing the IOM's recommendations have been made since the report was released in October of 2010. An infrastructure was created to advance the implementation of these recommendations (RWJF, 2011a): The Future of Nursing: Campaign for Action, is coordinated through Center to Champion Nursing in America (CCNA), an initiative of AARP, the AARP Foundation and the Robert Wood Johnson Foundation (RWJF). As a result of the Campaign for Action, action coalitions comprised of nurses and other health care providers, academic and philanthropic leaders, policymakers, businesses, and consumer advocates have been developed at a national level, as well as in 48 states (as of May 2012) throughout the country, to work on specific aspects of the recommendation (Future of Nursing: Campaign for Action, 2011). Additionally, the Senate Appropriations Committee has requested that Kathleen Sebelius, Secretary of the Department of Health and Human Services, develop a plan to implement the IOM recommendations and report back to the committee. Numerous other programs that aim to improve nursing education and increase the pipeline have also resulted (RWJF, 2011b).

One of the major themes of the IOM report The Future of Nursing (2011) is ensuring diversity. In fact, the IOM report illustrates diversity in all its forms, showcasing nurses from varied demographic backgrounds (e.g., geography, gender, race, and ethnicity), levels of educational preparation (e.g., BSN, MSN, DNP, and PhD), and practice settings (e.g., acute, primary, and community) in case studies throughout the report. The case for gender, racial and ethnic diversity was specifically addressed in recommendations number four and five. Although some examples of what is being done to increase the pipeline and diversity of nurses are provided in the report, it is clear that more needs to be done to bring these exemplary programs to scale. Additional efforts are needed to engage Hispanic nurses as part of the solution to advance health for all and specifically for Hispanic populations in the U.S. In the subsequent section, we highlight the implications of the IOM Future of Nursing (2011) report for Hispanic nurses and provide recommendations that could be employed to ensure that Hispanic nurses are an integral in efforts to lead change and advance health.

## Implications for Hispanic Nurses

### Education

Four of the eight IOM recommendations (i.e., recommendations 4, 5, 6, and 7) call for changes in the way that nurses are educated. Implementing these recommendations would require increasing the pipeline of Hispanic nursing students, especially in BSN, graduate, and doctoral programs. Currently only six percent of BSN students are Hispanic (National League for Nursing, 2011). Only 11 percent of nurses that are Hispanic report having received master's or doctorate degrees (U.S. Department of Health and Human Services, Health Resources and Research Administration, 2010). Consequently, Hispanics continue to be vastly underrepresented in the RN workforce, especially among Advanced Practice Registered Nurses (APRN) and PhD educators and scientists. As recommended in the report, programs are urgently needed that recruit Hispanics into nursing, ensure their retention, promote their progression onto higher levels of education, and encourage them to take faculty positions.

**Increasing the proportion of Hispanic BSN students.** Barriers to increasing the proportion of Hispanic BSN students have been previously described (Grumbach, Coffman, Gandara, Munoz, Resenoff , & Sepulveda, 2003; Sullivan Commission on Diversity in the Healthcare Workforce, 2004). Graduation from subpar secondary schools, inadequate career counseling, and the high cost of baccalaureate education are some barriers that, while not unique to Hispanics, disproportionately affect them. Conversely, successful elements, including mentoring, strengthening family and peer support, and financial and academic support (for sciences and English language skills), have been identified as integral to successful programs to recruit, retain, and graduate Hispanics in nursing. While there are several successful programs highlighted throughout this book, evidence-based programs that can be scaled up and sustained are needed to increase the proportion of Hispanics entering nursing.

One successful program that could be replicated and scaled up was implemented by the University of Texas El Paso School of Nursing (UTEP-SON). The program aimed to increase the number of Hispanic nursing students from economically disadvantaged backgrounds and ensure that these students passed the National Counsel Licensure Examination-Registered Nurse (NCLEX-RN) exam on their first trial (Anders, McInnis, Edmonds, Monreal, & Galvan, 2007). Various strategies were employed including a number of pre-nursing activities managed by an outreach manager who was a Hispanic male health professional and described as a "role model." These activities included outreach in three local high schools (e.g., field trips and summer orientations at UTEP-SON, faculty and student presentations), as well as outreach to the local community college. The program also offered financial and social support to nursing students through Project ARRIBA (Advanced Retraining and Redevelopment Initiative in Border Areas), a university-based program that provides support to economically disadvantaged Hispanic students. Students engaged in a number of mentoring and academic coaching activities that aimed to retain students and ensure their success (e.g., monthly meeting with a case manager). The project resulted in a 25 percent increase in the number of students from Hispanic and other racial/ ethnic minority backgrounds. Further, all the graduates from this program have passed the NCLEX-RN on their first attempt (Anders et al., 2007). The success of this program provides support for the development of programs in other areas of the country where a high proportion of Hispanics reside. Like the program at UTEP-SON, programs should target students at various stages in their academic trajectory (i.e., high school, community college, and university) as well as provide a combination of financial and social support. More programs that incorporate similar approaches need to be developed and evaluated.

Since the majority of Hispanic nurses, for various financial and access related issues, enter nursing through community colleges, articulation programs to increase the number of BSN graduates are needed. While many programs are focused on the individual, strategies are also needed between BSN and ADN programs to ensure a seamless transition. Community college-university partnership programs are a promising strategy to increasing the proportion of nurses with a BSN to 80 percent. One exemplar is the Oregon Consortium for Nursing Education (OCNE), a partnership between eight community colleges and the Oregon Health and Science University School of Nursing (OCNE, 2012). This partnership shares a common curriculum that allows associate's degree earning nursing students who are enrolled in the community college to be dually enrolled at the university. Once students complete the ADN portion of the program, they are able to complete their BSN degree without having to apply to the university or leave their home communities.

The OCNE model has resulted in a student population that is more likely to continue onto obtaining their BSN (45 percent) and more likely to be comprised of minority students (OCNE, 2012). This type of model is ideal for Hispanic nursing students whom often have strong family ties that prevent them from leaving their communities. Since community colleges tend to have a more diverse student body than universities, community college-university bridge programs also hold promise in recruiting Hispanic and underprivileged students who would not have opportunities to attend the university due to financial barriers. Additionally, research supports the idea that nurses in general, not only Hispanic nurses, are more likely to work close to the nursing programs they attend (RWJF, 2010). Community college and university partnerships of these kinds need to be established throughout the country, especially in areas where large Hispanic populations reside.

**Doubling the number of doctorally prepared Hispanic nurses.** The lack of an adequate pool of Hispanic nurses prepared at the BSN level is a major barrier to increasing the proportion of graduate Hispanic nurses. The IOM Future of Nursing report (2011) recommends the development of bridge programs that facilitate the progression of RNs into graduate studies in nursing, especially doctoral degrees (e.g., BSN to PhD, MSN to DNP). Many different types of bridge programs have sprung up throughout the country in the past decade. For example, Loyola University in New Orleans has a program that they describe as the BLEND MSN bridge. This program allows a student with a non-nursing bachelor's degree to enter the MSN program by completing a six-credit "bridge" which includes required undergraduate courses (Loyola University, 2010). As of fall 2010, there were 65 schools offering similar MSNs to non-nursing graduates (American Association of Colleges of Nursing [AACN], 2012). The University of Washington School of Nursing has a program that allows RNs with a BSN to obtain a PhD with or without completing the MSN along the way (Williams, 2007). As of fall 2010, there were 73 schools offering similar BSN to PhD programs (AACN). Nevertheless, these programs do not seem to be attracting sufficient racial and ethnic minority nurses to reach the goals set forth in the IOM report. Barriers and facilitators that exist for entry into nursing and BSN programs are similar for progression into PhD and graduate programs. Importantly, the number of doctorally prepared Hispanic nurses is small, thus making exposure to Hispanic role models difficult at best.

Highlighting both challenges and strategies confronted in increasing the number of Hispanics graduating from PhD programs are efforts undertaken at the University of Miami School of Nursing and Health Studies (UMSONHS). While UMSONHS is located in Miami-Dade County, which has a Hispanic majority (65 percent) (U.S. Census Bureau, 2012), and is the second most diverse private research university in the country (after Howard University), minorities are still underrepresented compared to the local community. For example, 30 percent of the doctoral students are Hispanic, none of whom come from their BSN to PhD program. This is somewhat lower than the 34 percent of Hispanic students in the BSN program, indicating that Hispanic nurses are less likely to progress on to doctoral education. To increase the proportion of Hispanic students enrolled in their PhD program, UMSONHS is in the process of creating bridge programs with universities in other areas of the county (e.g., Miami Lakes, which is 81 percent Hispanic) and country (El Paso, which is 81 percent Hispanic) where there are large numbers of Hispanic BSN students (U.S. Census Bureau). The program will minimize cost and the time students have to spend away from their families and communities through eliminating summer breaks and using technologies (i.e., in the case of the El Paso students). UMSONHS is developing other strategies aimed at taking away the "cold," non-family oriented, and intimidating atmosphere often associated with research institutions and creating a warmer more supportive environment so that Hispanic PhD students feel supported. Nursing has been at the forefront of providing culturally specific care for Hispanics. This same commitment and know-how needs to be transferred to the development and evaluation of strategies that aim to engage Hispanic nurses in doctoral education.

## Leadership

The IOM Future of Nursing report (2011) recommends that nurses be prepared to assume a wide array of leadership positions. While few in number, Hispanic nurses have a legacy of leadership. In government, for example, Henrietta Villaescusa was the first Hispanic nurse to be appointed as health administrator, Health Services Administration, Department of Health, Education and Welfare, and the first Mexican-American chief nurse consultant in the Office of Maternal and Child Health, Bureau of Community Health Services. Recently, Patricia Montoya served as the director of Health and Human Services for the state of New Mexico and also as the director for the Agency for Children, Youth, and Families at the Department of Health and Human Services. Rose Gonzalez MPS, RN has served as director of government affairs at the American Nurses Association. Sara Gomez Erlach, a public health advocate, worked tirelessly to develop and advocate for migrant farm workers in California. She drafted the proposal that established 75 federal rural health clinics, which led to the creation of additional state clinics. She was also the first woman to receive the rank of full colonel in the history of the U.S. armed forces.

The impact of these Hispanic nurses is evident on local and national health policy and also highlights the important bridge that Hispanic nurses span between nursing and Hispanic communities. Importantly, Hispanic nurse leaders are emerging at the bedside, community, state and federal levels, and in the public and private sectors across the spectrum of nursing education, practice, and research. As we work to develop leaders, it is important that Hispanic nurses also be prepared to function well in both Hispanic and nursing venues (see Box 2.2). An important component of Hispanic nurse leadership is Hispanic cultural knowledge, awareness, and skills (including bilingual abilities), as well as connection to communities. A distinguishing component of Hispanic nurse leadership is reflected in comments by noted sociologist David Hayes-Bautista (Learning to Give, n.d.):

Look for your passion and follow it ... but do it from a Latino perspective, where you are guided by the effect of what you do on your family and your community. Being Latino is emotional, is spiritual, and to me it means moral structure: what is good, what is right, what is just.

Expanding opportunities for Hispanic nurses to lead. The IOM Future of Nursing report (2011) recommends that health care organizations, academic institutions, governments, and other health organizations provide opportunities for nurses to be part of collaborative teams and lead efforts in coordinating patient care, conducting research, redesigning health care delivery systems, and diffusing innovative practices. Nevertheless, Hispanic nurses face barriers to lead. For example, a recent article published in Science reported racial and ethnic disparities in the likelihood of obtaining R01 level funding from the National Institutes of Health (NIH) (Ginther et al., 2011). The disparity in research funding limits the potential that Hispanic researchers have in creating evidence-based practice that may benefit their communities. Similarly, the U.S. Office of Personnel Management (OPM) (2011) reported that only eight percent of the permanent federal workforce was Hispanic. Further, while the presence of other minorities had risen in recent years, there was much smaller growth among Hispanics. This limits the ability of Hispanic nurses to shape the implementation of health policy and government-sponsored health programs.

Organizations involved in addressing health care issues in the U.S. should assess the opportunities for leadership they are providing to Hispanic nurses and be held accountable for developing, implementing, and evaluating plans of actions for increasing these opportunities. For example, in response to the under-representation of Hispanics in the federal workforce, the OPM launched the Hispanic Council on Federal Employment. This council is charged with developing strategies to recruit, retain, and promote Hispanics in government positions (OPM, 2012). It is important that this council and similar responses by organizations consider the importance of promoting Hispanics, especially nurses, in health-related leadership positions as a means of ensuring that the populations they serve are more accurately represented. Success stories of how nurse-led initiatives have resulted in eliminating health disparities among vulnerable urban and rural communities (RWJF, 2011c) provide evidence to support the potential impact that Hispanic health leaders can have on improving the health of the communities they come from.

Preparing nurses to lead. For Hispanic nurses to create the changes in the health care delivery system that are needed to address health inequities, they need to be prepared to be leaders. The responsibility of this preparation lies not only within the academic institutions that educate nurses, but also with their employers, professional organizations supporting Hispanic nurses, and Hispanic nurses themselves. Hispanic nurses need to commit themselves to leading health and health care at both the bedside and board room levels. For Hispanic nurses to be effective in their commitment, they need to acquire skills in nursing research, health policy, management, interdisciplinary collaboration, and communication. While there are a number of national leadership programs that exist for nurses and Hispanics, Hispanic nurses do not take advantage of these opportunities, are not prepared or supported through the selection process, and for other reasons, are underrepresented. These leadership competencies are often not part of the standard ADN curriculum and Hispanics are more likely to enter nursing through the ADN route, articulation agreements between community colleges and universities are particularly important for increasing the capacity of a more diverse RN workforce that is ready to lead.

In addition to ensuring higher levels of education of Hispanic nurses, current nursing programs need to improve the effectiveness of their leadership curriculum across all levels (i.e., BSN to doctoral) and develop ways to ensure this competency is developed. Simulation appears to be a promising approach for teaching and evaluating leadership (Reed, Lancaster, & Musser, 2009). However, many of the academic settings where

Hispanic nursing students attend may not have access to state-of-the-art simulation. Innovations for teaching leaders should be expanded (e.g., virtual simulation) to increase the access that Hispanic nursing students have to leadership learning opportunities.

Mentorship is another key strategy in preparing nurses to lead. For Hispanic nurses to want to be leaders, they need to be inspired and mentored by others who have been effective in creating positive changes in health care and health. An exemplary mentorship program is the National Coalition of Ethnic Minority Nurses Associations' (NCEMNA) Scholars Program. NCEMNA is a coalition of five ethnic minority nursing organizations (Asian American/Pacific Islander Nurses Association, National Alaska Native American Indian Nurses Association, National Association of Hispanic Nurses, National Black Nurses Association, and Philippine Nurses Association of America) that supports ethnic minority researchers at all career levels and engages ethnic minority students to consider nursing research as a career trajectory (NCEMNA, 2012). In the Scholars Program, nursing students interested in research are paired with a national mentor who has demonstrated leadership in research in a similar topic area (e.g., HIV prevention targeting Hispanics). Mentees are sponsored to attend a national conference where they meet their mentor and work with their mentor during the conference and well after on clearly established research and leadership goals. Institutional and national mentorship programs that connect Hispanic nurses with leaders in their areas of research, teaching, and practice should be created and expanded to allow junior Hispanic nurses to benefit from the wealth of experiences of nurse leaders who have been effective in creating positive changes in nursing, health care, and health.

### Table 2-2
Recommended Strategies for Advancing the Future of Nursing for Hispanics

**Education**

- Recruitment efforts aiming to attract Hispanics into nursing need to begin early at the high school level and continue throughout the different educational levels and settings (i.e., technical schools, community colleges, and universities). Special attention should be given to schools that serve a large proportion of Hispanic students. Recruiters should have characteristics that potential nursing students could identify with (e.g., having a similar background) and serve as role models.

- Programs that provide financial and social support (e.g., case management) for underprivileged students should be provided through schools of nursing.

- Community college and university partnerships facilitating the seamless progression of students from the ADN to BSN educational levels need to be established throughout the country, especially in geographic areas where there is a high proportion of Hispanic residents.

- Programs that provide bridges for nursing students to obtain master's and doctoral degrees need to develop strategies that appeal to and are sensitive to the academic and cultural needs of Hispanic students.

**Leadership**

- Organizations involved in addressing health care issues in the U.S. should assess the opportunities for leadership they are providing to Hispanic nurses and develop, implement, and evaluate plans of actions for increasing these opportunities.

- Nursing education needs to improve the effectiveness of its leadership curriculum and develop ways to ensure this competency is developed and evaluated. Innovative methods for teaching and evaluating leadership (e.g., simulation) need to be developed, evaluated, and made available to Hispanic student nurses.

- Hispanic nurses should influence the future of nursing and health care by making sure they are present at decision-making tables, sharing their unique perspectives, drawing upon their support structures (e.g., family) to be more effective leaders, and saying yes to opportunities to have an impact, even when this is uncomfortable.

# CONCLUSIONS

**Summary of Required Transformation**

Hispanic nurses will need to be engaged in redesigning the health care delivery system for a growing Hispanic population. This will require that the number and capacity of Hispanic nurses be dramatically increased. The IOM report on the Future of Nursing (2011) provides a blueprint for achieving this. We recommend key strategies that will facilitate progress towards these goals (see Table 2.2). First, more Hispanics need to graduate from BSN programs — either through direct entry into a BSN program or through rapid and seamless progression from ADN to BSN. Second, a greater proportion of Hispanic nurses must progress on to graduate education, especially doctoral education. Third, academic institutions, health care organizations, governments, and other health organizations need to develop strategies to ensure that influential positions are filled by competent Hispanic nurse leaders. Lastly, Hispanic nurses need to develop competencies that will facilitate their success as leaders, and leadership programs in nursing and health care need to ensure inclusion of Hispanic nurses.

**Box 2-1 Reflections by a Hispanic Nurse Committee Member on the IOM Report on the Future of Nursing (2011)**

When I was contacted by the leadership of the initiative on the future of nursing regarding participating on the IOM Committee on the Future of Nursing, I was terrified. What could I, a young and inexperienced Hispanic nurse faculty, possibly contribute to the future of nursing? I felt a weight on my shoulders — a responsibility for shaping the future, a responsibility for which I felt I was not ready. Nevertheless, I did what most nurses do when called upon. I signed up for the extra shift.

**Lesson 1: Believe that you belong at the decision-making table.**

During the first meeting, I quickly figured out that I was a little different than everyone else. First, I was one of just five nurses on the 18-member committee. I was the only Hispanic nurse and one of two Hispanic females on the committee. I was also much younger and less experienced than everyone else. I recall reviewing the other committee members' biographical sketches ahead of time, being impressed with their accomplishments, and feeling like I did not belong at the table. Nevertheless, I quickly became aware of the value I brought to the table. As the only young Hispanic nurse faculty, I had unique expertise and experience that was needed. With this realization, I began to build the courage to share my perspectives with the committee. Although not always in agreement, my perspective was always valued. I learned that everyone has something to contribute. Do not turn down decision-making opportunities because you do not feel worthy of them.

**Lesson 2: All you have to do is contribute one thing that is important to have an impact. Do what it takes to have this one contribution heard.**

I decided to follow the advice of a great Hispanic nurse leader and mentor who told me that the only thing I had to do to be successful is make one meaningful contribution during every committee meeting. This recommendation did not only help minimize my feelings of intimidation, but also provided me with guidance on how to plan my contributions. Every meeting I made sure to read everything that was sent to me and prepared myself to express one important point regarding the future of nursing. Sometimes I would even rehearse what I wanted to say. I did not speak often, but when I did, I spoke to issues that I knew a great deal about. It was not always easy to be heard. When you are at the table with a group of leaders, it is often hard to get a word in. Nevertheless, I began to use some of the tactics used by other committee members. I did not always wait to be called upon to speak and sometimes I even interrupted others when they spoke. At the end of the process, I really felt that I had an impact. Much of the content and recommendations of the IOM report relating to population health, health disparities, nursing education, and diversity were influenced by the contributions I made during these meetings. I would have never imagined that I could have such an impact.

**Lesson 3: The Hispanic family is not a barrier to leadership, it is a facilitator. You do not have to choose between your family and work. You can have both.**

When asked to be on the IOM Committee on the Future of Nursing, I was pregnant with my first son. My first reaction to agreeing to serve on the committee was that of guilt. I questioned whether I could be a good mother now that I had agreed to attending meetings, traveling, and spending a good portion of my extra time on helping to shape the future of nursing. What about the future of my son and family? However, I quickly figured out that my family did not interfere with my ability to serve on the committee, but rather allowed me to do so more effectively. For example, three months after my son was born, my father traveled with me and the baby to the National Academies of Sciences in Washington, DC. My father brought the baby to me during lunch and breaks so I could breastfeed and still be back in time to contribute to the committee process. There are countless other examples where the support of my family helped me be in a better position to contribute to the committee, whether it was by allowing for me to practice how to communicate my ideas to the other committee members more effectively, bringing me food when I was tired, or providing me with the balance I needed in life to be more effective professionally.

**Lesson 4: It is in the extra shift where you can have the biggest impact. Say yes as much as you can, especially when it is uncomfortable.**

There were many opportunities to do extra work, both during the development of the IOM report and after its release. Although I was intimidated by some of the tasks involved in these opportunities, I tried to say yes to as much as I could. The most uncomfortable of these opportunities was agreeing to be the spokesperson for Spanish-language media. It was hard enough feeling comfortable communicating to the committee in English, and I had agreed to communicate in Spanish to local and national audiences. My first interview was live on Despierta America, one of the most widely viewed shows on Univision, the largest Spanish TV network in the U.S. Needless to say, I was terrified. However, with the support from the RWJF, IOM, committee members, and family, I built enough courage to show up for the interviews. Although I participated in many, my nervousness never completed subsided. I would say this is a small price to pay for the opportunity to promote a greater future for nursing and health care.

## REFERENCES

American Association of Colleges of Nursing. (2012). Accelerated programs: The fast track to careers in nursing. *In American Association of Colleges of Nursing.* Retrieved January 27, 2012, from http://www.aacn.nche.edu/publications/issue-bulletin-accelerated-programs

Anders, R. L., McInnis Edmonds, V., Monreal, H., & Galvan, M. R. (2007). Recruitment and retention of Hispanic nursing students. *Hispanic Health Care International, 5*(3), 128-135.

Future of Nursing. (2011). *Future of Nursing – Campaign For Action.* Retrieved on July 6, 2012 from http://thefutureofnursing.org/about.

Grumbach, K., Coffman, J., Gandara, P., Munoz, C., Resenoff, E., & Sepulveda, E. (2003). *Strategies for improving diversity of the health professions.* Woodland Hills, CA: The California Endowment.

Institute of Medicine. (2002). *Unequal treatment: Confronting racial and ethnic disparities in health care.* Washington, DC: The National Academies Press.

Institute of Medicine. (2004). *In the nation's compelling interest: Ensuring diversity in the healthcare workforce.* Washington, DC: The National Academies Press.

Institute of Medicine. (2011). *The future of nursing: Leading change, advancing health.* Washington, DC: The National Academies Press.

Learning to Give. (n.d.). Quotes about Hispanic/Spanish/Latino. *In Learning to Give: philanthropy education resources that teach giving and civic engagement.* Retrieved on July 10, 2012 from: http://learningtogive.org/search/quotes/Display_Quotes.asp?page_num=2&subject_id=155&search_type=subject

National Coalition of Ethnic Minority Nurse Associations. (2012). Home. *In National Coalition of Ethnic Minority Nurse Associations.* Retrieved on January 31, 2012, from http://www.ncemna.org/

National League for Nursing. (2011). *Nursing student demographics 2008-2009.* In National League for Nursing. Retrieved from http://www.nln.org/research/slides/index.htm

U.S. Office of Personnel Management (OPM). (2011). *2010 Governmentwide Hispanic employment data.* Retrieved from http://www.opm.gov/diversityandinclusion/reports/hispanic/hispanicreport_sep2011.pdf

U.S. Office of Personnel Management (OPM). (2012). *Hispanic council on federal employment.* Retrieved from http://www.opm.gov/diversity/hispaniccouncil/hispanic_council_charter.pdf

Oregon Consortium for Nursing Education. (2012). *About OCNE.* In Oregon Consortium for Nursing Education. Retrieved on January 27, 2012, from http://ocne.org/

Pew Research Center. (2008). *U.S. population projections: 2005-2050.* Retrieved from Pew Research Center website: http://www.pewhispanic.org/2008/02/11/us-population-projections-2005-2050/

Reed, C. C., Lancaster, R. R., & Musser, D.B. (2009). Nursing Leadership and Management Simulation Creating Complexity. *Clinical Simulation in Nursing, 5*(1), e17-e21.

Robert Wood Johnson Foundation. (2010). *Distance between nursing education program and workplace for early career nurses (graduated 2007-2008).* Retrieved from the Future of Nursing website, a project of the Robert Wood Johnson Foundation: http://thefutureofnursing.org/NursingResearchNetwork5

Robert Wood Johnson Foundation. (2011a). *The future of nursing: Campaign for action.* Retrieved from the Future of Nursing website, a project of the Robert Wood Johnson Foundation: http://thefutureofnursing.org/about

Robert Wood Johnson Foundation. (2011b). *The future of nursing: Campaign for action. First year accomplishments.* Retrieved from the Future of Nursing website, a project of the Robert Wood Johnson Foundation: http://thefutureofnursing.org/highlights/detail/first-year-accomplishments

Robert Wood Johnson Foundation. (2011c). *Recommendation 2: Expand opportunities for nurses to lead and diffuse collaborative improvement efforts.* Retrieved from the Future of Nursing website, a project of the Robert Wood Johnson Foundation: http://www.thefutureofnursing.org/recommendation/detail/recommendation-2?quicktabs_1=1#quicktabs-1

Sullivan Commission on Diversity in the Healthcare Workforce. (2004). *Missing persons: Minorities in the health professions: A report of the Sullivan Commission on Diversity in the Healthcare Workforce.* Washington, DC: Author.

U.S. Census Bureau. (2012). *State and county quick facts.* Retrieved from http://quickfacts.census.gov/qfd/states/12/12086.html

U.S. Department of Health and Human Services, Health Resources and Services Administration. (2010). *The Registered Nurse Population: initial findings from the 2008 National Sample Survey of Registered Nurses.* Washington, DC: US. Government Printing Office.

Williams, D. (2007). *A faster path to the PhD.* Retrieved from Minority Nurse website: http://www.minoritynurse.com/bsn-phd/faster-path-phd

.

# CHAPTER 3
## FINDING AND KEEPING DIVERSITY IN YOUR PROGRAM: HISPANICS IN THE HEALTH PROFESSIONS

*Mary Lou Bond, PhD, RN, CNE, ANEF, FAAN*
*Carolyn L. Cason, PhD, RN*
*Pat Gleason-Wynn, PhD, RN, LCSW*
*Jennifer Gray, PhD, RN*
*Jean Ashwill, MSN, RN*
*Claudia S. Coggin, PhD, CHES*
*Michael D. Moon, MSN, RN, CNS-CC, CEN, FAEN*
*Elizabeth Trevino Dawson, DrPH, MPH*
*Michael Lopez, BA*
*Linda Denke, PhD, RN*
*Susan Baxley, PhD, RN*

The National Institutes of Health lists health disparities among vulnerable populations as one of the top five priorities demanding attention in the United States (Institute of Medicine, 2006). The Sullivan Commission on Diversity in the Healthcare Workforce (2004), in its much referenced report, cites the lack of minorities in the health professions as a major factor associated with the ever- increasing disparity in health among vulnerable populations. Efforts to prepare a health care workforce that is more culturally sensitive and competent such as those sponsored by the U.S. Department of Health and Human Services Office of Minority Health (2008) play an important role in improving health care for all, but do not address the central issue of diversity of the workforce as recommended by the Sullivan Commission on Diversity in the Healthcare Workforce.

Funded by the W. K. Kellogg Foundation, the Sullivan Commission on Diversity in the Healthcare Workforce (2004) gathered testimony from stakeholders across the United States to learn more about the underlying reasons for the lack of diversity in the health care professions. The year-long project yielded recommendations that included examination of and changes in the environments of health professions schools, improvements in the K-12 educational system, and commitments from leaders to increase diversity in their institutions.

The recommendations issued by the Sullivan Commission on Diversity in the Healthcare Workforce in 2004 provided the background and impetus for the study described in this chapter, in which Hispanics provided their views on the perceived institutional and personal barriers and the perceived supports needed for Hispanics in schools of nursing and public health in three universities in Texas.  The collective views of these Hispanics, along with the recommended best practices described in the literature, led to the development of the two self-assessment inventories described at the end of the chapter and included in Appendices B and C.

## BACKGROUND

Hispanics remain the fastest growing minority population in the U.S (U.S. Census Bureau, 2011). According to the Health Resources and Service Administration (HRSA) (2010), the proportion of Hispanic nurses between 2004 and 2008 increased from 2.3 to 3.6 percent. Further, an estimated 35 percent of the population in Texas is Hispanic (Texas Population Estimates and Projections Program, 2006). As cited by the Texas Statewide Health Coordinating Council (2011), the 2009 Board of Nursing licensure records estimates that only 11.3 percent of the nurse workforce in Texas is Hispanic. The 2011 Institute of Medicine (IOM) recommendations emphasize the need to increase the diversity of students to create a workforce prepared to meet the demands of diverse populations across the lifespan.

Hispanic high school students are less likely to enroll in a post-secondary education program than their white counterparts (Chapa & de la Rosa, 2006). Traditionally, Hispanics attend community colleges and fewer of them pursue advanced degrees (Anders, Edmonds,

Monreal, & Galvan, 2007). In fact, only 6.6 percent of all bachelor's degrees and 3.8 percent of all doctorates are awarded to Hispanics (Chapa & de la Rosa). According to Fry (2011), there has been a notable increase in the rate of Hispanic students enrolled in college from 13 percent in 1979 to 32 percent in 2009. Nursing schools ought to seize this opportunity to recruit Hispanic students to pursue nursing as a career to help care for the growing Hispanic population (Anders et al., 2007). Recruitment and retention efforts must be geared at eliminating financial, cultural, academic, social, and environmental barriers faced by Hispanic students (Anders et al., 2007).

The literature suggests that a major factor in a Hispanic student's choice to go to college, decision about where to go to college, and success in overcoming the challenges associated with completing a degree are very much influenced by the college's or university's openness to diversity (Rivera-Goba & Wallen, 2008). Cultural and racial isolation, lack of relevance of curriculum to minority issues, invisibility, and distance from program staff and faculty may contribute to stratified social relations. These factors can threaten the persistence and professional development of minority students (Daniel, 2007). According to Taxis (2006), Hispanic student success is enhanced when there are opportunities to build caring and bicultural affiliations within the institution. Therefore, faculty must seek to eliminate biased representations in classrooms, foster dialogue on race and ethnicity, and adopt curricula that can enhance multicultural understanding and competence (Maton et al., 2011).

Hispanic students are more likely to seek support from their mentors than are students from other ethnicities. For Hispanic nursing students, family and peer support is integral to their success (Ong, Phinney, & Dennis, 2006; Taxis, 2006; Torres Campos et al., 2009). Additionally, mentors are frequently viewed as part of the broad network of family members (Lynn, 2006). Student-centered programs and strong student services focused on giving students individual attention increase Hispanic students' success (Buchbinder, 2007). Student involvement in formal on-campus activities, including nursing student associations, contributes to greater satisfaction, greater academic success, and less likelihood of leaving school (Amaro, Abriam-Yago, & Yoder, 2006; Fischer, 2007). Providing a variety of success interventions including financial aid, access to academic coaches, participation in career fairs, and support services for social and economic issues are key elements that can aid Hispanic pre-nursing students to complete BSN programs (Anders et al., 2007).

There is a persistent pattern of low expectations for Latino/a students (Cavazos & Cavazos, 2010). Poor preparation and insufficient mentoring in K-12 and in undergraduate education is prevalent among Hispanics (Cavazos & Cavazos; Gonzalez, 2006). Low performance in developmental mathematics among Hispanics also means under-representation in the health care field (Rivera-Goba & Wallen, 2008). Other factors that contribute to attrition among minority students in nursing programs include family responsibilities, lack of financial resources, and lack of faculty (Rivera-Goba & Wallen).

According to Wilson, Andrews, and Leners (2006), institutional barriers that hinder ethnic participation in nursing include lack of faculty sensitivity to cultural differences, feelings of under-representation, institutional racism, cultural miscommunication, and lack of professional role models. Additionally, Latino students must often contend with major obstacles that impede academic success including the lack of financial, emotional, and social support resources (Alicea-Planas, 2009; Anders et al., 2007). When provided with the needed resources and formal mentoring programs designed to overcome their skill deficits, such students can become successful (Wilson, Sanner, & McAllister, 2010).

**Framework and Purpose of the Study**

The factors that support and/or impede Hispanic students' persistence in pursuing post-secondary education are captured, in part, in Valverde and Rodriquez's (2002) Model of Institutional Support. The model describes institutional barriers and supports for program completion among Hispanic doctoral students undertaking their studies at a Hispanic serving institution as financial support, emotional and moral support, mentorship, and technical support. For this study, the model was adapted in two ways. First, the literature suggests that advising is distinct from mentoring, so they were included in the adapted model as separate constructs. To make it more appropriate to education for professionals, the construct of professional socialization, the opportunity to do independent, creative work, linked with the opportunity to present these findings in a supportive professional environment (Conway, 1992), was added. The Adapted Model of Institutional Support as cited in Bond et al. (2008) is presented in Figure 3.1.

*Figure 3-1 Adapted Model of Institutional Support for Hispanic Student Degree, (Bond et al., 2008).*

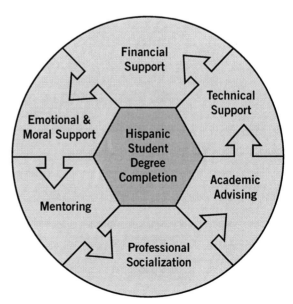

**Completion.** The adapted model served as the framework for studying the perceptions of Hispanic students enrolled in health professions programs. The study ascertained their perceptions of the barriers to persistence and their perceptions of the supports that facilitated persistence. The study also obtained the perceptions of members of Hispanic professional health organizations on their role in supporting students in the health professions.

## Study Participants, Setting, and Approach

Students in health professions programs (nursing and public health; n = 48) and health care professionals (n = 29) who self-identified as Hispanic participated in one of 12 focus groups. Student participants were enrolled in one of the following three institutions: (a) a Hispanic-serving, private liberal arts institution located in South Central Texas, (b) a state liberal arts institution, or (c) a state health science center. Both state institutions were located in North Central Texas. In each school of nursing, students participated in a focus group scheduled for their program: BSN (n = 14), RN to BSN (n = 8), MSN (n = 13), and PhD (n = 1). In the school of public health, both MPH and DrPH students participated in a single focus group (n = 12). A majority of the participants were age 20-29 (31 percent), married (64 percent), born in the United States (83 percent), and identified as Mexican American (78 percent; 83 percent female).

Members of Hispanic health professional organizations participated in focus groups scheduled for their organization, a north central Texas chapter of the National Association of Hispanic Nurses (NAHN; n = 11), a south central Texas chapter of NAHN (n = 9), and the Hispanic Health care Professionals Association (HISPA; n = 9; three of whom were nurses).

A Hispanic team member conducted each focus group by using starter questions generated from the Adapted Model of Institutional Support. The focus groups, which averaged an hour in duration, were audio recorded. One team member transcribed the audiotapes, and two other team members independently verified each transcription. A fourth team member completed a qualitative content analysis on each transcription, identified codes congruent and non-congruent with the model, and wrote a summary of findings that included interpretative comments with verbatim exemplars. The entire team reviewed these summaries, discussed their fit with the model, and discussed the meaning of themes that did not fit the model.

A detailed description of the study methodology and the study results is provided in Missing in Texas: Hispanics in the Health Professions – A White Paper (Bond et al., 2007). Views of undergraduate participants and members of health care professional organizations have been described by Bond, Gray, Baxley, Cason, Denke, and Moon (2008).

## Summary of Results

Collectively, the participants' comments supported previous findings reported in the literature. Examining participants' observations within the context of the framework of the study, however, not only organizes their reported experiences, but also helps to explicate their meaning as barriers or supports. For verbatim exemplars of each of the constructs of the model see Bond, et al. (2007) and Cason et al. (2008).

**Financial support.** Financial support is much more encompassing than paying for tuition and fees. Although the occasional participant benefited from adequate financial support from her/his family and university scholarships, the contingencies of most participants' lives included financial responsibilities associated with providing for their families; going to school added transportation and childcare costs. To meet these responsibilities they were employed. Having a job meant that they could not go to school full-time and, thus, were not eligible for university scholarships. The ways in which the participants and their families responded to managing debt were almost exclusively associated with gainful employment. Their lack of knowledge about opportunities for financial assistance as it relates to availability and accessibility and incurring and managing short-term debt in exchange for long-term gains compounded their challenges as students and family members.

To overcome the challenges associated with financial difficulties, participants' comments indicated need for support in (a) learning about ways to finance their educations, (b) finding funding opportunities, and (c) applying for funds. Although none of the participants directly suggested the need to revise the full-time requirements for scholarship eligibility, they did indicate that this requirement served as a barrier to getting needed support.

**Emotional and moral support.** For participants in this study, barriers related to emotional/moral support stemmed primarily from tension within their families emanating from their families' lack of understanding about their decision to go to college and their career choice. For some, inadequate support from faculty served as a barrier. Some voiced access to faculty as a problem, and others described faculty as insensitive to cultural differences. Health care professionals openly identified discrimination or racism as a barrier, as did students from two of the focus groups composed of graduate students. The centrality of emotional/moral support from one's family to success is evident throughout the participants' comments. A very close second source of emotional/moral support is that provided by peers, primarily classmates who were not necessarily from Hispanic backgrounds.

**Mentoring.** A major barrier associated with mentorship and the role it plays in helping Hispanic students succeed is an acknowledged absence of Hispanic role models in the health professions to serve as mentors. Their absence was especially noted among participants in undergraduate health professions programs. Non-Hispanics sometimes served in the role of mentor for these students, but they often evidenced a lack of knowledge about Hispanic cultural values, especially the role of family. Though participants indicated it would be ideal to have mentors who are Hispanic, they indicated mentors need not be Hispanic in background as long as they were grounded in Hispanic cultural values and beliefs. Respondents commented that mentors need to be caring individuals willing to help.

Having mentors helps students succeed, especially those seeking second degrees. In addition to faculty, some of the participants in this study referred to nurses, clinical preceptors, and family members who were health professionals as mentors. Participants from the health care professional organizations saw mentorship as one of their primary roles in helping students succeed. The participants from the professional organizations and those in graduate studies were less likely than undergraduates to express such concerns about non-Hispanic mentors.

**Academic advising.** The greatest barrier to persistence reported by students in undergraduate programs was the perceived absence of academic advising or the limited and non-responsive nature of academic advising when present. Health care professionals identified it as a barrier to both recruitment to and persistence in health education programs. They suggested the absence of such advising to students while they are still in high school precludes many from seeking entry into college and does not prepare them for the academic demands associated with college.

When academic advising is viewed positively, as it was by the graduate student participants, it serves as an important facilitator of student success. Comments from the undergraduate student participants suggested that academic advising entails more than course advisement. Their comments suggest that a more open, sustained interaction is needed to facilitate their success, and support that gets them beyond admission must be provided.

**Technical support.** Participants offered few comments related to either barriers or supports relative to technology. Access to computers prior to entry into college to learn about and apply for financial assistance was a problem for some, but once in college, participants reported they either had a personal computer or had ready access to one. Technical support services were noted to be readily available, as many of the classes used technology to deliver instruction, and on-line classes were considered supportive to success, especially for graduate students.

**Professional socialization.** For undergraduate participants, participation in activities related to professional socialization was limited. The major barrier to participation related to the time such activities were scheduled; they often conflicted with activities required for course completion, family responsibilities, or employment. Graduate student participants indicated that university activities were not as valued as were activities associated with professional organizations. Participants from health care professional organizations acknowledged the challenge of getting and keeping people involved. All participants commented on the desirability of involvement in professional activities, and greater involvement of professional organizations in mentoring and supporting students was seen as important to students' successes.

**Emergent Themes**

Bond et al. (2008) identified two additional themes that were not directly congruent with the Adapted Model of Institutional Support — self-determination and culture. Participants seeking second degrees and those in one of the professional organization groups identified self-determination as the way in which they overcame barriers to become successful. Comments related to culture were associated with valuing education, overcoming poverty, and moving into roles that departed from cultural expectation.

## DISCUSSION, CONCLUSIONS, AND RECOMMENDATIONS

An important limitation of this study is that the Hispanics in this study were predominately Mexican in origin and may hold different views and values than do other Hispanics who trace their ancestry to other countries. Although there was variability in the participants in terms of age, gender, socio-economic status, marital status, and first generation in college, the results do not necessarily generalize to all Hispanics in Texas or to all Hispanics.

The Adapted Model of Institutional Support served as a useful framework, at least in this study, for understanding and organizing Hispanic students' and Hispanic health care professionals' views of barriers and supports related to entry into and persistence in health professions education programs. Given these Hispanic participants' views, the definitions of each of the constructs included in the model need to be broadened to better reflect the Hispanics' prior experiences, personality, values, and attitudes. The construct definitions must reflect Hispanics' ethnic and social identity. As Lee (2006) pointed out, ethnic identity can be an empowering factor in student success and can be enhanced in environments that offer opportunities for ethnic expression and exploration.

Recruitment and persistence initiatives have increased the number of those in the nurse workforce from minority backgrounds. These increases, however, reflect the changing demographics of minority populations, but they are not closing the gap. In some settings, minority patients receive poorer quality of care than their white counterparts (Anders et al., 2010). Hospitals that have a high percentage of Spanish speaking and bachelor's prepared nursing staff demonstrate excellent outcomes of care (Anders et al., 2010). Thus, health professions programs and the institutions in which they reside must pursue more aggressive strategies to increase the percentage of individuals from minority groups who are attracted to their programs and must implement strategies that are known to help such students be successful in completing health professions programs. Such efforts are in line with Recommendation 4 of the IOM report (2011) — to increase the proportion of nurses with baccalaureate degrees who will "partner with education accreditation agencies, funders and employers to increase the diversity of students to create a workforce prepared to meet the demands of diverse populations" (p. 4). To support such efforts, two self-assessment inventories are offered to health professions programs and the institutions in which they reside to evaluate their recruitment and graduation initiatives.

The Institutional Self-Assessment for Factors Supporting Hispanic Student Recruitment and Persistence Tool developed by Cason, Bond, and Gleason-Wynn (2007); and the Healthcare Profession Education Program Self-Assessment developed by Gray, Bond, and Cason (2007a) are based on the findings of the study reported here and the recommended best practices described in the literature. The sections on the self-assessment tools are the constructs of the Adapted Model of Institutional Support and the items within each section reflect the broader definition of each construct and derive directly from the perspectives of Hispanics who participated in this study and as reported in the literature.

The self-assessment tools were later evaluated for validity and reliability in a National League for Nursing (NLN) funded study in 2010. Provosts, deans, and directors of nursing programs from eight states with high Hispanic populations and one of the authors of the initial Model of Institutional Support participated in the study. The item content validity associated with each construct/characteristic (CVI-I), ranged from 83 percent to 100 percent; reliabilities for the ISA and PSA for items ranged from .86 on the ISA and from .77 to .86 on the PSA. The validation process resulted in minor modifications in the tools. The revised tools are included in Appendices B and C.

In summary, the ISA and the PSA both hold strong psychometric properties and can serve as a basis for both institutions and programs to assess their environments and to establish benchmarks for improvements. It is through continued recruitment and retention of Hispanics into the nursing profession that health disparities will decrease for a growing majority of Hispanics.

## REFERENCES

Alicea-Planas, J. (2009). Hispanic nursing students' journey to success: A metasynthesis. *Journal of Nursing Education, 48*(9), 504-13.

Amaro, D. J., Abriam-Yago., K., & Yoder, M. (2006). Perceived barriers for ethnically diverse students in nursing programs. *Journal of Nursing Education, 45*(7), 247-254.

Anders, R. L., Edmonds, V. M., Monreal, H., & Galvan, M. R. (2007). Recruitment and retention of Hispanic nursing students. *Hispanic Health Care International, 5*(3), 128-135.

Anders, R. L., Bean, N. H., Fancher, D., Smead, D. G., Rosenthal, P. S., & Bader, J. O. (2010). An examination of disparities in a Hispanic-serving hospital using the agency of health care research and inpatient quality indicators. *Hispanic Health Care International, 8*(2), 107-115.

Bond, M. L., Cason, C. L., Gleason-Wynn, P., Denke, L., Gray, J., Ashwill, J., . . . Baxley, S. (2007). *Missing in Texas: Hispanics in the health professions – A white paper.* Arlington, TX: School of Nursing, University of Texas at Arlington.

Bond, M. L., Gray, J. R., Baxley, S., Cason, C. L., Denke, L., & Moon, M. (2008). Voices of Hispanic students in baccalaureate nursing programs: Are we listening? *Nursing Education Perspectives, 29*(3), 136-142.

Buchbinder, H. (2007). *Increasing Latino participation in the nursing profession: Best practices at California nursing programs.* Los Angeles, CA: The Tomás Rivera Policy Institute.

Cason, C. L., Bond, M. L., & Gleason-Wynn, P. (2007). *Institutional self-assessment for factors supporting Hispanic student recruitment and persistence.* Arlington, TX: School of Nursing, University of Texas at Arlington.

Cason, C. L., Bond, M. L., & Gleason-Wynn, P. (2010). *Institutional self-assessment for factors supporting Hispanic student recruitment and persistence (revised).* Arlington, TX: College of Nursing, University of Texas at Arlington.

Cason, C. L., Bond, M. L., Gleason-Wynn, P., Coggin, C., Trevino, M., & Lopez, M. (2008). Perceived barriers and needed supports for today's Hispanic students in the health professions: Voices of seasoned Hispanic health care professionals. *Hispanic Health Care International, 6*(1), 41-50.

Cavazos, A. G., & Cavazos, J. (2010). Understanding the experiences of Latina/o students: A qualitative study for change. *American Secondary Education, 38*(2), 95-109.

Chapa, J., & De La Rosa, B. (2006). The problematic pipeline: Demographic trends and Latino participation in graduate science, technology, engineering, and mathematics programs. *Journal of Hispanic Higher Education, 5*(3), 203-221.

Conway, M. E. (1992). The optimal environment for socialization of the nurse-scientist. *Nurse Educator, 17*(3), 24-27.

Daniel, C. (2007). Outsiders-within: Critical race theory, graduate education and barriers to professionalization. *Journal of Sociology & Social Welfare, 34*(1), 25-42.

Fischer, M. J. (2007). Settling into campus life: Differences by race/ethnicity in college involvement and outcomes. *The Journal of Higher Education, 78*(2), 125-161.

Fry, R. (2011). *Hispanic college enrollment spikes, narrowing gaps with other groups.* Retrieved from Pew Hispanic Center website: http://pewhispanic.org/reports/report. php?ReportID=146

Gonzalez, J. C. (2006). Academic socialization experiences of Latina doctoral students: A qualitative understanding of support systems that aid and challenges that hinder the process. *Journal of Hispanic Higher Education, 5*(4), 347-365.

Gray, J. R., Bond, M. L., & Cason, C. L. (2007a). *Healthcare profession education program self-assessment.* Arlington, TX: School of Nursing, University of Texas at Arlington.

Gray, J. R., Bond, M. L., & Cason, C. L. (2007b). *Healthcare profession education program self-assessment (revised).* Arlington, TX: College of Nursing, University of Texas at Arlington.

Health Resources and Services Administration. (2010). *The registered nurse population: Initial findings from the 2008 National Sample Survey of Registered Nurses.* Retrieved from Health Resources and Services Administration website:  http://bhpr.hrsa.gov/ healthworkforce/rnsurveys/rnsurveyinitial2008.pdf

Institute of Medicine. (2006). *Examining the health disparities research plan of the National Institutes of Health: Unfinished business.* Washington, DC: National Academies Press.

Institute of Medicine. (2011). *The future of nursing: Leading change, advancing health.* Washington, DC: The National Academies Press.

Lee, M. B. (2006). How and why ethnicity matters: A model for developing programs that serve students of color. In M. B. Lee (Ed.). *Ethnicity matters: Rethinking how black, Hispanic, and Indian students prepare for & succeed in college* (pp. 117-150). New York, NY: Peter Lang Publisher.

Lynn, M. R. (2006). Mentoring the next generation of systems researchers. *Journal of Nursing Administration, 36*(6), 288-291.

Maton, K. I., Wimms, H. E., Grant, S. K., Wittig, M. A., Rogers, M. R., & Vasquez, M. J. (2011). Experiences and perspectives of African American, Latina/o, Asian American, and European American psychology graduate students: A national study. *Cultural Diversity and Ethnic Minority Psychology, 17*(1), 68-78.

Ong, A. D., Phinney, J. S., & Dennis, J. (2006). Competence under challenge: Exploring the protective influence of parental support and ethnic identity in Latino college students. *Journal of Adolescence, 26*(6), 961-979. doi:10.1016/j.adolescence.2006.04.10

Rivera-Goba, M. V., & Wallen, G. R. (2008). Increasing the pipeline of Hispanic nurses: Are we making a difference. *Hispanic Health Care International, 6*(4), 170-171.

Sullivan Commission on Diversity in the Healthcare Workforce. (2004). *Missing persons: Minorities in the health professions: A report of the Sullivan Commission on Diversity in the Workforce*. Washington, DC: Author.

Taxis, J. C . (2006). Fostering academic success of Mexican Americans in a BSN program: An educational imperative. International *Journal of Nursing Education Scholarship, 3*(1), 1-14.

Texas Statewide Health Coordinating Council. (2011). 2011-2016 Texas state health plan. In *www.dshs.state.tx.us*. Retrieved on December 9, 2011, from http://www.dshs.state.tx.us/chs/shcc/reports/SHP2011-2016

Torres Campos, C. M., Phinney, J. S., Perez-Brena, N., Kim, C., Ornelas, B., Nemanim, L., . . . Ramirez, C. (2009). A mentor-based targeted intervention for high-risk Latino college freshmen: A pilot study. *Journal of Hispanic Higher Education, 8*(2), 158-178. doi:10.1177/1538192708317621

U. S. Census Bureau. (2011, May 26). *The Hispanic population 2010: 2010 census briefs*. Retrieved on November 28, 2011 from U.S. Census Bureau website: http://www.census.gov/prod/cen2010/briefs/c2010br-04.pdf

U.S. Department of Health and Human Services, Office of Minority Health. (2008, July 8). *Cultural competency*. In Initiatives. Retrieved on July 6, 2012 from http://minorityhealth.hhs.gov/templates/browse.aspx?lvl=2&lvlID=14

University of Texas at San Antonio. Institute for Demographic and Socioeconomic Research. Texas State Data Center. (2006). *Projections of the population of Texas and* counties in Texas by age, sex and race/ethnicity for 2000-2040. San Antonio: Texas State Data Center, The University of Texas at San Antonio.

Valverde, M. R., & Rodriquez, R.C. (2002). Increasing Mexican American doctoral degrees: The role of institutions in higher education. *Journal of Hispanic Higher Education, 1*(1), 51-58.

Wilson, A. H., Sanner, S., & McAllister, L. E. (2010). An evaluation study of a mentoring program to increase the diversity of the nursing workforce. *Journal of Cultural Diversity, 17*(4), 144-150.

Wilson, V. W., Andrews, M., & Leners, D. W. (2006). Mentoring as a strategy for retaining racial and ethnically diverse students in nursing programs. *The Journal of Multicultural Nursing & Health, 12*(3), 17-23.

# CHAPTER 4
## RETAINING HISPANIC STUDENTS IN BSN PROGRAMS

*Maithe Enriquez, PhD, RN, ANP-BC*
*Eve McGee, MSW*

Much emphasis has been placed on the critical need to recruit students from underrepresented ethnic minority groups, including Hispanics, into United States nursing programs (Gilchrist & Rector, 2007; Gordon & Copes, 2010; Williams, 2006). However, without effective strategies to enhance the success of these underrepresented students and the ability to support student professional development, such recruitment efforts can be futile. In this chapter, we describe successful strategies utilized to retain underrepresented minority students in the University of Missouri-Kansas City (UMKC) bachelor's of science in nursing (BSN) program. In particular, we focus on our endeavors with Hispanic students in an effort to give voice to the unique needs of this subgroup. We hope that our experience will be informative to other nurse educators and help them retain diverse nursing students in their programs.

## COMMITMENT TO DIVERSITY

The University of Missouri-Kansas City School of Nursing (UMKC-SON) was founded in 1979, and until 11 years ago, offered only professional degrees to registered nurses in the form of RN-to-BSN, MSN, and PhD programs. In 2000, the board of curators approved a pre-licensure Bachelor of Science in Nursing (BSN) degree program. UMKC-SON admitted its first BSN students in the fall semester of 2001 and became the first urban public university to offer a pre-licensure BSN program in Kansas City. From the onset of the BSN program, UMKC-SON made a commitment to recruit and graduate a diverse undergraduate student body.

### Barriers to Success for Minority Students

A number of barriers to college success have been identified for undergraduate students who are from underrepresented minority groups. Among these barriers are inadequate academic preparation at the high school level, limited high school career counseling, and a lack of financial support (Baron & Swider, 2009). Hispanic students often must work while in college to supplement family income, which can serve as a major barrier to success in college (Hood, 2010). In addition, the scarcity of nurse faculty and practicing nurses from underrepresented ethnic and racial groups leads to yet another barrier, a lack of diverse professional role models and mentors (de Leon Siantz, 2011).

**Risk for attrition.** Ethnic minority and first-generation college students are at higher risk for attrition than Caucasian students and students whose parents are college graduates (Ishitani, 2006). There are many factors, both academic and non-academic, that can contribute to high attrition rates for these students, and factors contributing to attrition can exist in tandem or in isolation from one another. Academically, when students are not prepared for college due to inadequate high school preparation, students struggle with basic survival skills such as time management, and study and note-taking skills. As a result, students often spend extra time studying and preparing for classes, often become overwhelmed, and fall behind in their coursework. Consequently, feelings of self-doubt, shame, and fear of failure cause students to doubt their decision to obtain a degree. For some students, non-academic challenges can also leave them feeling overwhelmed. Balancing work, school, and family can be difficult and financial constraints can make having a job necessary. Hence, little time is spent on schoolwork resulting in poor grades. Early recognition of these risk factors can serve as signals and help to identify students who may be at risk for academic failure or who intend to withdraw from school (Reason, 2009).

**Underrepresented minority BSN students at UMKC-SON.** Since its inception, UMKC-SON has consistently reported an enrollment of 25 to 27 percent ethnic minority students in the BSN program. For the fall semester 2007, of the 215 students enrolled at UMKC-SON, 27 percent were from African-American/black, Hispanic, and Asian backgrounds. In addition, approximately 30.5 percent of these students were first generation college students. Hence, since 2002, UMKC-SON has implemented a variety of intervention programs to address retention of underrepresented undergraduate students. In this chapter we describe UMKC-SON's experiences and lessons learned over the past five years as we have evaluated and refined our retention programs and strategies (see Table 4.1).

### Retention Programs

At our school of nursing, the primary pipeline for ethnic minority student recruitment is the Kansas City, Missouri, public school system. This school system has faced a number of academic challenges over the past two decades, including loss of accreditation. In an effort to better understand the specific needs of ethnic minority and low-income prospective students from this pipeline, UMKC-SON conducted focus groups with high school students from the Kansas City, Missouri, public school system in 2001. Focus group participants were African-American, Hispanic, Caucasian, Native American, and Asian low-income high school students. Participating students were asked what would help them pursue a college education and a career in nursing. Students identified family support as the number one factor that would help in both aspects. In addition, students also identified (a) services received from social service agencies such as physical/mental health services, employment assistance, and food; (b) academic support; (c) financial support; (d) self-control and self-confidence; (e) transportation; and (f) housing support as factors helping them obtain a college education. Female students also identified child care as something that might help women in the pursuit of a college education. We used the information gained from these focus groups to inform our retention strategies and develop our programs.

We implemented four programs and strategies from 2002 to 2011 that directly impacted Hispanic students — Nursing FIRST, targeted Spanish-language marketing,

Nursing Workforce Diversity, and Social Work Case Management. The most successful strategies from these four programs were then refined and implemented as the Student Success Program, our current comprehensive retention program. The Nursing Workforce Diversity and the Social Work Case Management programs remain in place.

**Nursing FIRST.** Nursing FIRST (Forming Relationships for Support), a two-year pilot project that aimed to enhance retention and develop the leadership skills of undergraduate pre-nursing students from underrepresented minority groups, was our first formal retention program. A two-year grant was secured from a local foundation to provide staff time, program materials, and light refreshments for students during program sessions. The program targeted freshmen and had two components — mentoring and academic support.

*Mentoring support.* The mentoring component provided a faculty, alumni, or community nurse member of like ethnic background and similar nursing interests, such as pediatrics, as a mentor for the undergraduate student. Mentors were volunteers recruited from the UMKC-SON alumni association and local chapters of professional nursing organizations such as the Black Nurses Association, National Association of Hispanic Nurses, and Sigma Theta Tau. Many community and alumni members had indicated an interest in mentoring a student, and several had participated in the taskforce meetings to develop the program. Mentor training provided an overview of mentor responsibilities, expectations, boundaries of the mentor/mentee relationship, and strategies to engage the student mentees. Training was provided by a minority nurse with expertise in pipeline and mentoring programs. The Nursing FIRST project staff matched students with trained mentors.

Students participated in the Nursing FIRST mentoring component on a voluntary basis and were encouraged to meet at least monthly during the freshman (pre-nursing) year with their mentors. Mentoring activities included shadowing, visits to the mentor's health care setting, one-on-one meetings, communicating by phone, and email communication. Mentors encouraged students to also participate in the Nursing FIRST activities that were designed to help students achieve academic success.

*Academic support.* The second component of the Nursing FIRST program encompassed supplemental instruction and academic prep sessions in targeted areas. Prep sessions were advertised on the school's website and on bulletin boards in the schools. While prep sessions were open to all students, the Nursing FIRST staff targeted underrepresented students and encouraged their participation through individual letters and personal phone calls from Nursing FIRST staff. In addition, undergraduate faculty members were asked to identify underrepresented students who were struggling in their coursework and refer these students to the Nursing FIRST staff for possible participation in the program. The Nursing FIRST academic prep sessions included math (algebra), power point and presentation skills, medical terminology, test-taking skills, and writing skills for English language learner (ELL) students. Sessions were offered monthly on a rotating basis and were facilitated by Nursing FIRST staff, volunteer faculty, and volunteer mentors. Students requiring more extensive academic support were referred to UMKC's Supplemental Instruction program, an international model for student academic assistance (Malm, Bryngfors, & Morner, 2011).

Students in the Nursing FIRST mentoring component and those referred by faculty, because the student was perceived to be struggling academically, received additional advising. One additional advising session was added prior to the midterm of each semester. During the advising session, the students' current grades and success to that point were discussed and changes or need for additional support identified. The additional session offered an opportunity to refer students for supplemental instruction and academic or other types of support early in the semester. The School of Nursing established a detailed database to capture retention data, which tracked student participation, maintained continuity of information among staff members, and collected program evaluation data.

***Nursing FIRST outcomes.*** An average of 13 students attended each academic prep session (range two to 25 students). Students were asked to complete an evaluation form at the end of each session. The majority (94 percent) of students indicated that the sessions were helpful. Over the two-year period of the program, only one student ever indicated that he/she did not find a session valuable. Of the 11students who participated in the mentoring component (four Hispanics, two Asians, and five African Americans), 100 percent were retained.

Reaching Hispanic parents through Spanish-language marketing. Just over 10 percent of our undergraduate students were of Hispanic descent, and some were first-generation immigrants whose parents preferred the Spanish language. Our school's experience working with Hispanic students had indicated that their parents generally had played a vital role in their lives, a relationship which the university had not always recognized. In 2002, with funding from a small internal grant, and with the collaboration of UMKC's communications department, we created a brochure in Spanish to reach these parents. The content was designed, edited, and reviewed by professional Spanish-language experts, the school's bilingual faculty members, and Hispanic community advisors, resulting in a two-color brochure. The brochure explained potential careers in nursing and provided information on UMKC, the SON, and available financial aid. We continue to use this brochure.

**Nursing Workforce Diversity (NWD) program.** In 2003, UMKC-SON was awarded a grant by the U.S. Department of Health and Human Services, Health Resources and Services Administration (HRSA) to support the Nursing Workforce Diversity (NWD) program, which addressed the need for more culturally diverse nurses. The NWD program addressed retention issues by providing financial, academic, and social support to students considered to be disadvantaged, including racial and ethnic minorities underrepresented in nursing, enrolled in the BSN program.

Students determined to have the highest financial need, based on data from annual applications for federal financial aid, participated in the NWD program. The HRSA grant, together with $450,000 in fundraising by UMKC-SON, provided $3,000 each year in stipends to a total of 80 students for four years. The stipends allowed students to concentrate on their education, reduced financial stressors, and decreased, or in some instances eliminated, the need to work.

NWD program participants were required to participate in mentoring either by a nurse in the community or mentoring by an upperclassman. Students were paired with mentors and asked to interact monthly with mentors via e-mail, phone, or in person. Initially, mentoring was well received by students, especially if the mentoring relationship served an immediate need such as obtaining information from an upperclassman about a particular course or instructor. However, over time the daily demands and rigor of the nursing program made it difficult for students to devote the necessary time and energy required to maintain a viable mentor-mentee relationship.

The NWD students also received academic advising from faculty who had received additional training about how to assist disadvantaged students. Academic advisors developed plans of study for students on an individual basis, factoring in the results of their Test of Essential Academic Skills (TEAS), which measured readiness in math, science, reading, and English. In addition to the TEAS, students underwent an assessment of writing and computing skills to determine the need for additional preparation prior to admission into the nursing program. The NWD students also received an additional academic advising session prior to the midterm of each semester when there was still time to identify struggling students with problem areas such as low grades. Then necessary students were referred to supplemental instruction, UMKC's writing lab, UMKC's math lab, and other tutorial opportunities. The additional advising meeting per semester provided additional academic support referrals and also served as a relationship-building experience.

***Nursing Workforce Diversity (NWD) program outcomes.*** Outcomes for the students who participated in the NWD program were encouraging. Of the 80 students who participated, 85 percent were retained. Nine NWD participants were Hispanic; all but one were retained. An exit survey completed by the Hispanic student who dropped indicated that the student had personal issues that resulted in her inability to stay in school, specifically, the need to work and care for her children, ages two and four.

**Table 4-1  Retention Strategies Targeting Underrepresented BSN Students 2002-2007**

| Program/ Intervention | Year began/ended | Major Components | Funding Source(s) |
|---|---|---|---|
| Nursing First | 2002-2004 | Mentoring by community nurses; Academic prep sessions | Foundation grant |
| Spanish-language marketing | 2002 to ongoing | Brochure targeting parents | Internal university diversity grant |
| Nursing Workforce Diversity | 2003 to 2006 | Stipends for students with high financial need; Mentoring by upper-classmen; Additional advising | HRSA Endowed fund |
| Social work case management | 2004 to ongoing | Counseling; Life skills | HRSA Foundation grant |
| Student Success Program | 2006 to ongoing | Supplemental instruction; ELL support group; Emergency financial assistance; Critical thinking intervention | UMKC-SON budget item; Private donations; Foundation grant |

**Social work case management.** In response to the high need for social and emotional support by undergraduate nursing students, UMKC-SON initiated case management services in 2004. The addition of a master's-prepared social worker to the faculty was initially made possible through funding from the Prime Health Foundation and later sustained by the SON and other grants. The National Association of Social Workers (NASW) (2007) defined social work as a profession that helps individuals, families, and groups change behaviors, emotions, attitudes, relationships, and social conditions to enhance their ability to meet personal and social needs. Social work interventions, such as case management, are innovative approaches to nursing student retention, by which a social worker assists students with a wide variety of long- and short-term men¬tal, emotional, behavioral, and environmental challenges. Such challenges include marital and family difficulties; adjustments related to balancing school, work and family; or alcohol and substance abuse. As a result, students can optimize their overall functionality, which enhances academic success.

In addition to the common financial and academic needs of undergraduate students, UMKC-SON underrepresented minority nursing students were also found to experience problems with housing, childcare, employment, and mental health. Together these problems posed significant barriers to their success in the undergraduate nursing program. The social worker has been able to identify significant needs within this student population. Students had lived within environments with poor secondary education, widespread poverty, violence, substance use, and homelessness. As these students entered the nursing program, they brought the effects of these problems with them.

The following are actual cases which the social worker has encountered with Hispanic students:

*Case 1.* Maria was a 31-year-old female who had experienced several recent losses and was referred by a faculty member to the social worker. Maria expressed trouble eating and sleeping and drastic changes in behavior, withdrawal from friends and social activities, and a lack of interest in work and school. The social worker explored with Maria the possibility of suicidal ideation, which the student acknowledged. The social worker immediately developed a safety plan with her and set up a phone conference with the university psychological counseling center to further assess and manage the situation. The student received counseling services and was able to effectively deal with her stressful situations and completed her degree with confidence.

*Case 2.* Gabriela was a 23-year-old student with a four-year old son. The student had been living with her parents and was suddenly asked to immediately move out, leaving her with no place to live. The social worker referred the student to the housing authority and then discussed possible alternate living situations, along with employment possibilities. The social worker suggested ways to help the student adjust to taking care of her son alone. The student temporarily lived with a friend for approximately six months until she ultimately received public housing. During this time frame, the student began receiving child support and working part-time at a local retail store. The student stated that she would not have known how to handle her situation and without the intervention of the social worker would likely have dropped out of school.

*Case 3.* Angela, a 25-year-old student and single parent, experienced problems with child care, which was very stressful. The social worker helped the student locate a safe child care agency, encouraged her to explore flextime options with her employer, helped her with time management skills, and provided an intervention to help the young mother deal with the immediate stress of raising a child alone. Angela felt that the social worker's assistance allowed her to continue pursuing her BSN degree and focus on her educational goals.

*Case 4.* Lola, a 30-year-old mother of an eight-year-old son, had been dating her boyfriend for approximately one year when the relationship with the boyfriend turned violent. The student services office referred the student to the social worker who assessed the situation and determined that Lola was in an unsafe environment. The social worker contacted a domestic violence shelter and temporarily relocated the student. The social worker helped her make a safety plan that allowed her to move to the shelter. The assistance of the social worker helped the student realize that she had the ability to access services and resources that ultimately helped her stay in school.

There are many other examples of personal struggles and challenges that have put Hispanic students at risk for attrition in our nursing program. Students who have experienced personal challenges, such as lack of child care and unstable housing, were at great risk for academic failure because their focus shifted to immediate personal problems and away from educational endeavors. Over the past four years the social worker has provided services to students through assessment, conflict mediation, and resiliency building. Moreover, the social worker has provided referrals for prevention, routine intervention, and crisis intervention for suicide, substance, and alcohol problems.

In addition to interventions for personal problems that required immediate attention, the social worker has also helped students enhance their self-esteem, coping skills, and decision-making skills. The social worker has identified students in need of such services through referrals from the faculty. The social worker has offered to meet with these students on a weekly basis to process both negative and positive situations the student has encountered in the past week. These interactions with students have led to student-identified coping strategies and enhanced critical thinking and decision-making skills. Students identified challenges, strengths, and potential solutions and coping strategies, such as exercise and meditation. Finally, students who have been able to identify their challenges and visualize solutions to these challenges have successfully increased their coping and their overall self-esteem. These services were based in the social work strengths perspective, which strengthens an individual's ability to function competently, even in the presence of major life stressors (NASW, 2007). Working in collaboration with school psychologists, school counselors, school faculty, and administrators, the social worker integrated these resources to provide social, emotional, behavioral, and adaptive functioning support to students, the student's family, and the faculty.

*Social work case management outcomes.* Students (N = 52) were surveyed to examine satisfaction with social work case management services. The majority (75 percent) of students were satisfied with the social work services received and believed that interaction with the social worker was helpful. Most (83 percent) stated that they would refer a peer with a problem to the social worker. Of the students who were not satisfied with the social worker services, the majority commented that the social worker was not able to meet his/her needs due to a high demand for the social worker's services by other students, which resulted in a feeling that the social worker did not have time for them. As a result, our school added another part-time social worker to our staff. The following quote sent to the social worker via email illustrates the impact of such intervention on a Hispanic student's life:

I was a pre-nursing student a couple of years back and spent a lot of time working one-on-one with you during that year in learning how to juggle self care in my personal life with the expectations and learning curve of nursing life. I saw your name in my contacts and it prompted this email. I just wanted to **thank you** for all of the time, encouragement and resources that you invested in me. Your contribution was quite significant and I'm very grateful to have had that opportunity. I'm very excited and I'm looking forward to the journey that lies ahead. (E. Salazar, personal communication, February 21, 2006)

### Student Success Program

Our school's first four years of experience culminated in the Student Success Program, a comprehensive program that aims to increase the retention of underrepresented ethnic minority students in the BSN program. The Student Success Program was developed based on the evaluation and refinement of our past retention strategies. The program includes academic, social, and financial support and has the following five key components that directly impact the success of Hispanic students: case management, supplemental instruction, ELL support group, emergency assistance, and the critical thinking enhancement intervention.

*Case Management,* an essential component of the Student Success Program was discussed in detail earlier in the chapter and continues in its same format.

*Supplemental Instruction* (SI) is a specialized tutoring program for students enrolled in courses identified as high risk courses. High risk courses are defined as those courses with a higher rate of drop-out by underrepresented students, as compared to majority students. The SON financially supports SI for two courses: freshmen chemistry and sophomore pharmacology. SI sessions are held weekly to review content and concepts taught the previous week. Evaluation data has indicated that participants in SI, on average, have a 0.5 letter grade higher than those of nonparticipants. SI is an academic support program that was developed at UMKC, has been validated by the U.S. Department of Education, and has been replicated internationally (Malm, Bryngfors, & Morner, 2011).

The UMKC SI model of student academic assistance helps a student master content while developing and integrating learning and study strategies. The goals of SI include (a) to improve student grades in targeted courses, (b) to reduce the attrition rate within those courses, and (c) to increase the eventual graduation rates of students. All students in a targeted course are urged to attend SI sessions, and students with varying ability levels and ethnicities participate. There is no remedial stigma attached to SI, since historically difficult courses rather than high-risk students are targeted. Students participating in SI within the targeted nursing courses earn higher mean final course grades than students who do not participate in SI, regardless of ethnicity and prior academic achievement.

For students whose first language was not English, including Spanish-language dominant Hispanic students, unique challenges surrounding acquisition of the English language and American culture existed. This population of students often expressed difficulty with reading and comprehending texts, resulting in such issues as the need to read assigned chapters twice to better understand the content. In addition, these students had difficulty understanding the cultural nuances of the English language, medical terminology, and some health care concepts. Hence, the ELL support group evolved in response to the unique needs of ELL students. The ELL support group meets with native English-speaking students who attend and serve as peer tutors for ELL students. Students meet once a month and discuss academic and acculturation issues, in addition to successes and challenges in particular courses. Because developing fluency in English takes practice, ELL students are encouraged to talk in small informal settings and practice their communication skills to gain confidence in their English-speaking ability. The school social worker facilitates the group sessions and the ELL students also work one-on-one with the social worker monthly to improve note taking, study, and test taking skills. Informal feedback from ELL support group participants has indicated that students feel the group is beneficial.

Another situation that surfaced as a barrier to retention for Hispanic and other underrepresented students was unanticipated financial problems. Students voiced difficulty staying in school when unexpected financial constraints arose and they were unable to pay for rent, utilities, groceries, or other essential living expenses. As a result, emergency assistance is provided to students through a UMKC-SON fund supported by private individuals who contribute an undisclosed amount of money each year to the SON through anonymous donations. The fund can be used to assist students with unexpected expenses that occur during the academic year. Support is provided on a case-by-case basis for requests such as for assistance with food, medication, and transportation. Students with urgent financial need submit a letter asking for assistance and a committee of three SON staff members determines an amount of money to be awarded to the student. The fund has helped a number of Hispanic students stay in school.

One such example was a Hispanic female student who over the course of several months, noticed problems concentrating and focusing on everyday tasks. Her grades were beginning to decline and she was having trouble focusing on lectures, interacting with peers, and maintaining the motivation to get out of bed every day. The student, after referral to the UMKC Counseling and Testing Center by the school's social worker, was diagnosed as having a mood disorder and was prescribed medication. However, because the student had no prescription drug coverage, she experienced difficulty paying for her medication. At the time, the student was living with her mother, whose only source of income was Supplemental Security Income and $150 in food stamps a month. The student was awarded $500 from the emergency assistance fund to pay for her mental health medication and she was able to stay in school.

The final component of the Student Success Program is the Critical Thinking Enhancement Intervention, which began as a pilot program with the goal of enhancing critical thinking skills of sophomore students in two courses, Nursing Fundamentals and Adult Health I. Attrition patterns together with individual interviews with underrepresented students had indicated that success in these two courses was critical to progression in the nursing curriculum. The critical thinking enhancement program consisted of weekly sessions that lasted 90 minutes. Students' learning styles were identified, which allowed tailoring of skill building activities, and the sessions focused on content presented to students in Fundamentals and Adult Health I classes the prior week. Retention of course content was enhanced using questions modeled after the nursing licensure (NCLEX) exam. The goal of this program was to intervene while the student was still experiencing success, so that the foundation for the development of critical thinking skills could support subsequent coursework. Students were referred to the program by faculty, or students could self-refer to the program. Faculty members were encouraged to refer students at-risk for failure (i.e., if the student experienced a grade of 70 percent or less on an exam). The pass rate for students who participated in the intervention for Nursing Fundamentals and Adult Health I was 83 percent, compared to a 78 percent pass rate the year before the intervention was implemented. The critical thinking intervention continues for these two courses and plans are underway to expand this intervention to other courses.

### Implications for Retaining Hispanic Students

Over the past few years, UMKC-SON has learned a number of valuable lessons and now has a deeper understanding about the unique retention needs of Hispanic students. Hispanic students, in particular, benefit from mentoring by community nurses and faculty of like ethnic background and are quite amenable to mentoring relationships. The benefit is enhanced for Hispanic ELL students if the mentor speaks Spanish. Financial stress can be devastating for Hispanic students who tend not to seek loans or financial aid. We have found that Hispanic students need more guidance and encouragement to apply for scholarships and financial aid than our Caucasian and other underrepresented students. Few Hispanic students are aware of the opportunities for financial assistance, perhaps because many of our Hispanic students are first-generation college students and the children of immigrants. Because the family is very important to Hispanic students, we encourage any opportunity to involve the student's family/significant others in the BSN educational process.

Also critical to the retention of Hispanic students is early assessment and intervention. If academic and non-academic problems can be identified, addressed, and resolved early, then, in our experience, the risk for attrition can be reduced. Early intervention requires that faculty members be keenly aware of the need to recognize a potential problem and refer students for help at the first sign of an academic or non-academic problem. Hispanic students need to be aware of available services and coached to seek such services when problems arise.

In addition to the formal retention programs that we have previously discussed, several other informal retention strategies for Hispanic students exist that we feel have merit. These include: (a) direct interaction with faculty members, (b) exposure to Hispanic nurse mentors/preceptors, and (c) participation in the local chapter of the National Association of Hispanic Nurses (NAHN). Our faculty members involve Hispanic students in targeted research and clinical experiences in an effort to provide mentoring and leadership opportunities. For example, in a violence prevention intervention study implemented among Hispanic high school students, the research assistant is a bilingual/bicultural Hispanic sophomore BSN student who was in need of a part-time job that was flexible around her course and clinical schedule. In addition, faculty place Hispanic students in agencies with Hispanic nurses for their clinical experiences as assignments permit. Hispanic students are also encouraged to participate in the local chapter of the Hispanic Nurses Association.

Finally, our Hispanic faculty member invites Hispanic students to lunch or dinner at least once per semester and our dean provides funding for the meal expense. Students have commented that this informal interaction with faculty has resulted in feeling supported, cared about, and encouraged to explore graduate education. In addition, students welcomed the opportunity to speak their first language, Spanish, with a faculty member and other Hispanic students without fear of judgment.

**Lessons learned.** Our school's retention programs were refined based not only on formal evaluation, but also by our challenges. We learned that mandated mentoring was not effective. Hence, we now offer only volunteer mentoring opportunities to our students through activities such as placing Hispanic students in clinical settings with Hispanic nurses and interaction with Hispanic faculty, such as the lunches and dinners described above. We changed our financial assistance to a case-by-case emergency basis, rather than scheduled stipends, giving more opportunity for utilization of the resources for urgent and crisis situations. Instead of waiting until students are struggling, we now target underrepresented students for supplemental instruction and academic support in courses with a history of high drop-out rate by underrepresented students.

Above all, our school has found that having an experienced social worker available to students who are faced with personal challenges is a key strategy in our ability to retain Hispanic students. A professional who is certified to provide counseling services and can intervene before a problem becomes insurmountable can often prevent drop-out. Having a social worker on our staff has been an important learning experience which has provided much of our understanding about the positive impact that a social worker can have on Hispanic and other diverse student retention.

## CONCLUSIONS

While retention of Hispanic and other underrepresented students can be a challenge, the beneficial results for recipients of nursing care certainly justify the effort required. Given the current critical shortage of nurses from underrepresented minority groups, formal retention programs such as those described in this chapter are essential if nursing is to successfully address the lack of diversity in our health care workforce. A more diverse nursing workforce will contribute to enhanced health outcomes for diverse Americans and decrease health disparities (Institute of Medicine, 2011; Sullivan Commission on Diversity in the Healthcare Workforce, 2004).

## REFERENCES

Barton, A. J., & Swider, S. M. (2009). Creating diversity in a baccalaureate nursing program: A case study. *International Journal of Nursing Education Scholarship, 6*(1). doi:10.2202/1548-923X.1700

Gilchrist, K., & Rector, C. (2007). Can you keep them? Strategies to attract and retain nursing students from diverse populations: Best practices in nursing education. *Journal of Transcultural Nursing, 18*(3), 277-285.

Gordon, F. C., & Copes, M. A. (2010). The Coppin Academy for pre-nursing success: A model for the recruitment and retention of minority students. *ABNF Journal, 21*(1), 11-13.

Hood, L. (2010, October 29). *Unique challenges for Latino community college students*. Retrieved from the Hechinger Report website: http://hechingerreport.org/content/unique-challenges-for-latino-community-college-students_4485/

Institute of Medicine. (2011). *The Future of nursing: Leading change, advancing health*. Washington, DC: The National Academies Press.

Ishitani, T. (2006). Studying attrition and degree completion behavior among first-generation college students in the United States. *Journal of Higher Education, 77*(5), 861-885.

de Leon Siantz, M. L. (2011, fall). *Building capacity: A blueprint for faculty diversity*. Retrieved from Minority Nurse website: http://www.minoritynurse.com/building-capacity-blueprint-faculty-diversity

Malm, J., Bryngfors, L., & Morner, L. (2011). Supplemental instruction: Whom does it serve? *International Journal of Teaching and Learning in Higher Education, 23*(3), 282-291.

National Association of Social Workers. (2007). Webpage. In *National Association of Social Workers*. Retrieved on July 6, 2012 from http://www.socialworkers.org/nasw/default.asp

Reason, R. (2009). Student variables that predict retention: Recent research and new developments. *Journal of Student Affairs Research and Practice, 46*(3), 482-501.

Sullivan Commission on Diversity in the Healthcare Workforce. (2004). *Missing persons: Minorities in the health professions: A report of the Sullivan Commission on Diversity in the Healthcare Workforce*. Washington, DC: Author.

Williams, S. (2006, September 11). *Opening doors — Hispanic schools reach out to Hispanic students*. Retrieved from the Nurse.com website: http://news.nurse.com/apps/pbcs.dll/article?AID=2006609110408

# CHAPTER 5

## CONTRIBUTING FACTORS AND STRATEGIES TO ADDRESS THE SHORTAGE OF HISPANIC NURSING FACULTY

*Evelyn Ruiz Calvillo, DNSc, RN*

According to the American Association of Colleges of Nursing (AACN) (2011), data from member schools indicate only 12.6 percent of the nation's nursing educators are people of color. The shortage of ethnically diverse faculty is a problem that is complex (National League for Nursing, 2010). Schools of nursing are facing the challenge to recruit a diverse faculty and concurrently the challenge to retain the small pool of faculty. Recruiting eth¬nically diverse faculty into higher education has seen minimal progress in the percentages of full-time nursing faculty. Within the higher education community, myths and misconceptions affect the recruitment of ethnically diverse faculty. For example, it is often claimed that potential applicants are unqualified or unavailable. Such myths, stereotypes, and assumptions have helped maintain the status quo and have created significant barriers to increasing the number of Hispanic faculty.

Increasing the number of ethnically diverse faculty into nursing programs has been an issue for many years. There have been some changes in the number of faculty reported; however, there have been very subtle increases in the number of Hispanic faculty. In the last edition of this chapter, published over a decade ago (Calvillo, 1996), factors identified as contributing to the low numbers of Hispanic nursing faculty were the low wages and the number of Hispanic students entering nursing. Unfortunately, the number of Hispanic students entering nursing is still impacting progress. In recent years, other factors have become the focus of many public and private entities interested in increasing not only Hispanic nurses but also Hispanic faculty. The same issues impacting nursing in general, such as the aging and retiring of the current nursing workforce and not enough young people entering the profession, are affecting the shortage of Hispanic faculty. As time has passed, other factors have been identified contributing to this gap between supply and demand, such as the institutional environment and attrition rates. Many experts believe that increasing the participation of minorities is a key component in addressing the nursing shortage, and certainly filling the educational pipeline is one answer. Nursing as a career choice has yet to make an impression on the fast-growing Hispanic youth population. To do so would positively impact the number of Hispanic faculty in the future. Several strategies that were identified in the previous edition of Hispanic Voices (Calvillo) to increase Hispanic faculty still have relevancy today.

## CONTRIBUTING FACTORS TO SHORTAGE OF HISPANIC FACULTY

While the number of persons from ethnic minorities is increasing in the general population, the health care workforce continues to be largely homogeneous. Although initiatives have been undertaken or sponsored by the U.S. Department of Health and Human Services Office of Minority Health (2008) to prepare a more culturally sensitive and competent workforce, others have called for diversifying the workforce itself. In either instance, it is important to consider some key factors that are contributing to the shortage of Hispanic faculty.

## Low Number of Hispanic Nurses Prepared to Teach

The most significant factor is the low number of Hispanic nurses who are prepared to teach at learning institutions. Hispanics represent one of the largest, least-educated ethnic groups in the United States (Chapa & de la Rosa, 2006). The Pew Hispanic Center (2009) reported Hispanic high school students are less likely to enroll in a postsecondary education programs than their white counterparts. Nearly nine in ten (89 percent) Latino young adults ages 16 to 25 say that a college education is important for success in life; yet only about half that number (48 percent) plan to get a college degree. Hispanics accounted for only 12.8 percent of all public high school graduates. Although 82 percent of Hispanic high school seniors with college qualifications went on to college compared to 89 percent of white high school graduates, many Hispanic high school graduates tend to delay enrollment and are likely to choose two-year institutions (Pew Hispanic Center, 2009).

Nursing education's challenge to meet the needs of a more culturally diverse generation of students is compounded when there just is not enough culturally diverse faculty. The low number of stu¬dents who continue into graduate education in preparation for teaching is consistent with the severe shortage of minority nursing faculty that persists today. Many youth who begin postsecondary education at community colleges do not complete bachelor's degrees (Long & Kurlaender, 2009). Hispanic community college students significantly trail white peers in finishing bachelor's degrees. Less than 13 percent of Hispanic students who begin at community colleges complete a bachelor's degree, compared to 23 percent of their white peers. Less than 25 percent of Hispanic community college students finish a bachelor's or transfer to a four-year college, compared to 36 percent of white community college students. It seems that as educational level increases, the number of Hispanics who remained in college to graduation decreased, accounting for only 6.6 percent of all bachelors' degrees and 3.8 percent of all doctorates awarded (Chapa & de la Rosa, 2006). Studies have shown that 43.1 percent of Hispanic students receive their nurs¬ing degrees at the associate level. 2.1 percent of Hispanic nurses are prepared at the master's level and only 0.1 percent of Hispanic nurses have earned doctorates (U.S. Department of Health and Human Services, Office of Minority Health, 2008).Only 10.3 percent, overall, had a master's or doctoral degree. With only 7 percent of enrollment in baccalaureate programs, 5.1 percent enrollment in master's programs, and 4.7 percent enrollment in doctoral programs (AACN, 2012), it is difficult to increase the potential Hispanic faculty pool.

## Educational Pipeline of Hispanics into Nursing

Perhaps the most critical factor affecting the number of potential His¬panic faculty is the low enrollment of Hispanic students into nursing. Research indicates that the under-representation of minorities among faculty is largely an educational pipeline issue (American Association of State Colleges and Universities [AASCU], 2006). While nurses who reported they were Hispanic increased between 2004 and 2008, from 2.3 percent to 3.6 percent of the total number of RNs in the U.S. (U.S. Department of Health and Human Services, 2010), the number of potential faculty is still greatly affected. Although many nursing schools have slightly increased the racial and ethnic diversity of their student populations, the number of Hispanics entering nursing remains low (AACN, 2012 U.S. Department of Health and Human Services, 2010). The numbers in no way are representative of the patient population or the United States as a whole (Buchbinder, 2007). As the population of the United States continues to diversify, the failure of nursing to attract minorities into the profession will further exacerbate existing shortages as workers are drawn from a smaller and smaller part of the potential workforce. Several factors have contributed to the low number of Hispanics seeking nursing as a profession — (a) institutional policies regarding recruitment of Hispanics, (b) limited educational preparation in high school, (c) limited financial resources, (d) a dearth of Hispanic faculty and mentors to provide positive role models for nursing, and (e) the disproportion of Hispanic RNs to the Hispanic population (Sullivan Commission on Diversity in the Healthcare Workforce, 2004).

### Cultural Mismatch Between Hispanic Students and Educational Institutions

An important question regarding diversification is whether there is a real and meaningful rationale for changing the status quo of a teaching institution. Cultural traits and skills of ethnically diverse students are different than the mainstream U.S. culture. Villarruel, Canales, and Torres (2001) found that Hispanic women value pursuing education, but that family expectations often conflict with their personal values. Barriers related to emotional and/or moral support stem primarily from tension within their families emanating from their families' lack of understanding about their decision to go to college and their career choice. This cultural mismatch can lead to failure to achieve academic success (Pacquiao, 2007). Modification of a nursing pro¬gram through the hiring of diverse faculty who can relate to students from the same culture does appear to offer an answer to a complex issue.

Matching a diverse student population is now a key variable in recruiting diverse faculty into nursing programs. Demand for change has been influenced by the ideals and val¬ues that an ethnic mix of students brings to educational institutions. In many institutions, demands by ethnic groups are made through involve¬ment in governance or by demand for changes in the classroom. In some instances, demands are made by public protest. Additionally, as many state and federally supported educational institu¬tions are faced with potential cutbacks in dollars, serving the customer (i.e., the diverse student) has become important. As the numbers of ethni¬cally diverse students entering colleges or universities increase, institutions are also concerned about serving and, most importantly, satisfying the cus¬tomer by the earning of a degree.

To encourage more Hispanics to pursue nursing as a career, schools must be sensitive to the academic and cultural needs of the students (Peragallo, 2003). Hispanic students are particularly at risk of becoming lost in the academic world. Minority students often have difficulty with transition from the associate's to the baccalaureate degree and from the master's to the doctorate degree (Sullivan Commission on Diversity in the Healthcare Workforce, 2004). The typ¬ical college or university campus may be an unfamiliar social and aca¬demic situation, often comprised of predominately white undergraduates, faculty, and staff. The situation is complicated by the fact that many Hispanics enter college with poor language and reading skills, often due to inept preparation in high school. Continuation of their education is affected as well by economics.

Another contributor to the low numbers of Hispanic nurses is the attrition rates of students admitted into nursing programs. Students often view retention as the responsibility of the teaching institution (Wilson, Andrews, & Leners, 2006). Having access to successful role models, among other services provided by the institution, is key to motivate student success and leads to enhanced customer satisfaction. However, the dearth of Hispanic faculty and mentors to provide positive role models for Hispanic nurses in particular, impacts the success of programs that have well-intended goals.

## Impact of Growth of Hispanics in the U.S. on Supply of Hispanic Nurses

Perhaps the most ubiquitous force leading to change is the rapid growth rate of Hispanics in the United States. Many states may experience increases in the number of post-secondary degrees, but still may fall behind with respect to educational attainment if their general populations are growing faster because they are experiencing out-migration of educated citizens, or if growth is occurring disproportionately among particular groups. As the fastest growing minority population in the United States, Hispanics are expected to increase from 50.5 million to 132.8 million by the year 2050 (U.S. Census Bureau, 2011, August). By 2080, over half (51.1 percent) of the nation's population is predicted to consist of Hispanics. The health of the U.S. population depends on an adequate supply of health care providers — that is, nurses and a nursing workforce — that reflects the racial and ethnic composition of the population. The nurse population increased from 7.2 percent in 1980 to at least 12.2 percent in 2008 (U.S. Department of Health and Human Services, 2010). Hispanic or Latino RNs still remain the most underrepresented group of nurses when compared with the representation in the United States population (Sullivan Commission on Diversity in the Healthcare Workforce, 2004). After adjusting for those Hispanic or Latino RNs who provided no response to the question on race, only 3.6 percent of the RN population is Hispanic or Latino (U.S. Department of Health and Human Services, 2010), although Hispanics or Latinos comprise 16 percent of the general population (U.S. Census, 2011, March). Changing demographics and increasing diversity of the population of the U.S. are trends influencing the future of nursing education.

The AACN (2012) reported that the minority nursing student population increased from 21 percent in 2002 to 27.5 percent in 2011. Increases are attributed to national efforts to recruit and retain minority nursing students (Davidhizar & Shearer, 2005). However, the number of Hispanic nurses remains disproportionately small compared to the growth in the Hispanic population. Hispanics comprise less than two percent of all registered nurses (RNs) in the United States, and they are the least likely of any ethnic group to enter the nursing workforce with a baccalaureate degree (U.S. Department of Health and Human Services, 2010). Hispanic Americans are the second-largest and fastest growing minority in the United States yet Hispanics are seriously underrepresented in nursing programs at all levels.

Health care providers and related organizations in areas where His¬panic populations are growing are ever more concerned with enabling nurses and other health care professionals to provide culturally sensitive care to this large group. Culturally sensitive care is given when the provider considers and incor¬porates culture and ethnic beliefs into care, as well as health promotion based on diseases specific to racial and ethnic differences. Treating and educating patients about health promotion based on cultural considerations and beliefs can lead to a faster and better recovery. One solution here is to provide health care providers from the same ethnic or cultural group. Unfortunately, while health care organizations are recruiting Hispanic nurses intensely, the prospect of attractive ben¬efits and security in an uncertain job market often leads to postponement of plans to continue further education.

## STRATEGIES TO ADDRESS THE FACULTY SHORTAGE

By addressing the contributing factors, policy makers, educators, and members of the health care industry can help to increase the participation of Hispanics in the nursing workforce. Federal and state governments, as well as private organizations, have all responded to the nursing shortage crisis with legislative bills, contracted studies and projects, privately-funded initiatives, and faculty loan repayment grants. Major themes include improving distribution of health professions workers in underserved areas and improving the representation of Hispanics and other minorities in the nursing profession. Funding specifically for increasing diverse faculty has been set aside by some state legislatures, private organizations, and foundations (AACN, 2008).

### Responding to a Call for Action

The Sullivan Commission on Diversity in the Healthcare Workforce (2004), a 16-member panel composed of leaders from the fields of health, business, higher education, and law, was charged with the task of gathering testimony from stakeholders across the United States to learn more about the underlying reasons for the lack of diversity in the health care professions. Funded by the W. K. Kellogg Foundation, the year-long project resulted in a series of policy recommendations intended to increase the number of minorities in the health professions. General recommendations were made for examination of and changes in the environments of health professions schools, improvements in the K-12 educational system, and commitments to increasing diversity from institutional leaders. Specific recommendations were made that would assist potential students to prepare for and gain admission to health professions schools and receive financial assistance when needed. Recommendations to assist health care workers to become more culturally sensitive and competent were also presented.

Teaching institutions continue to seek ways of increasing the number of ethnically diverse faculty. Many models or frameworks have been proposed or imple¬mented to address the issue of multiculturalism, either by changes in curricula to reflect diversity in society or to increase the numbers of ethnically diverse students in the different disciplines. Numerous recruitment programs, educational outreach, tuition assistance, retention models, and mentoring models have been suggested or implemented to increase the opportunities for the ethnically diverse stu¬dent to enter the health professions (Bednash, 2003; Gilchrist & Rector, 2007; Sullivan Commission on Diversity in the Health care Workforce, 2004).

Several institutions have implemented diversity plans, which include a variety of elements for recruiting and retaining faculty. Private and government stakeholders are increasingly becoming involved in supporting action to address the shortage of ethnically diverse nurses and, ultimately, faculty. AACN believes that health care providers and the nursing profession should reflect and value the diversity of the populations and communities they serve. At the policy level, AACN recommends that stakeholders provide incentives and funds to schools of nursing to recruit faculty from diverse populations, increase scholarship funding for minority students pursuing advanced education, promote faculty careers to underrepresented groups, and engage minority faculty in the recruitment of students from their respective communities. Other actions include removal of financial barriers that prevent minority students from pursuing a nursing education, support for mentoring programs and targeted outreach programs launched by baccalaureate and higher degree schools of nursing, increased funding for Diversity Workforce Grants which are available through Title VIII of the Public Health Act, and raising the cultural competency level of all nurse educators and clinicians. Additionally, it is important to support community-based collaborations among educators, human services organizations, businesses, practice settings, and a wide range of stakeholders interested in enhancing cultural diversity in the health professions and providing needed services to the community (Bednash, 2003).

Federally supported models have concentrated on increasing the ethnically underrepresented health profes¬sion workforce who can provide primary health care.

Funding from the division of nursing, health organizations, and private foundations has in¬creased the number of graduates who can practice in various areas, al¬though little impact has been made in increasing the number of Hispanics with a master's or doctorate degree. Few, if any, models, projects, or programs have addressed the recruit¬ment and retention of ethnically diverse nurses who are prepared to con¬sider faculty appointments.

A systematic, comprehensive model for the recruitment and hiring of full-time underrepresented faculty into health occupations programs has been proposed by several institutions of higher education. Valverde and Rodriquez (2002) developed the Model of Institutional Support to describe institutional barriers and supports for program completion among Hispanic doctoral students undertaking their studies at a Hispanic serving institution. The model included the following four constructs: (a) financial support, (b) emotional and moral support, (c) mentorship, which included academic advising, and (d) technical support. Several groups supported by both private and government funding such as AACN, 2008; and the Sullivan Commission on Diversity in the Healthcare Workforce, 2004 have provided a forum in which specific strategies could be identified to increase the pool of underrepresented master's prepared can¬didates for full-time positions in health occupations programs. Some programs have focused on identifying the benefits of a diverse faculty or by increasing the pool of diverse applicants, especially for full-time appointments in health occupations programs

**Strategies for Recruitment**

Recruitment and retention initiatives have increased the proportion of the nurse workforce from minority backgrounds. The increases, at best, reflect the changing demographics of the population; but they are not closing the gap. In other words, while there may a higher number of minorities in the nursing workforce, there is a growing gap between the percentage of Hispanics preparing to practice nursing and the percentage of Hispanics population The goal of many projects, initiatives, or programs is recruitment of ethni¬cally diverse faculty. The keys to success are recruitment, hiring, retention, and sensitizing current faculty and staff to the advantages of a diverse faculty. Another important consideration is the individual faculty candidate who is actively being recruited. The individual brings a diversity of values, beliefs, knowledge, attitudes, aspirations, and experiences both personal and which should be taken into con¬sideration when hiring

A successful model or program must have resources and sources for recruitment of faculty candidates which may come from (a) funding agencies, government agencies, and private enterprises that can provide financial aid for the development of recruitment programs targeting ethnically diverse faculty; (b) political and professional groups, such as the American Nurses Association and the National League for Nursing (2012), which can provide assistance with re¬cruitment and information such as statistical data and strategies; and (c) institutional support and commitment to increase diverse faculty.

Multiple methods to recruit faculty candidates include the following: (a) ca¬reer days; (b) ethnically sensitive printed materials, which include role models; (c) invitations of ethnic practitioners to conferences and work¬shops as participants and attendees; (d) relationships with ethnic or¬ganizations, especially for assistance with mentor programs; (e) marketing of the teaching role as a specialty; and (f) bridging with health agencies and graduate programs to provide teaching internships and to develop ad¬junct faculty positions for involvement in curriculum development and participation as guest lecturers (Taxis, 2006; Valverde & Rodriquez, 2002; Wilson, Andrews, & Leners, 2006). Bridge programs and seamless educational pathways offer opportunities for increasing the overall diversity of the student body and nurse faculty not only with respect to race and ethnicity but geography, background, and personal experience as well (Institute of Medicine, 2011).

**Action strategies for recruitment.** The process or the series of strategies are put into action beginning with recruitment strategies addressing the issues of ethnically diverse faculty. The following strategies are identified from various models, programs, and institutions cited in this chapter:

1. Respond immediately to letters of inquiry from potential candidates. Often candidates are discouraged by the slow response of many insti¬tutions. A good candidate may accept a position elsewhere if institu¬tions respond slowly. A quick response increases the candidate's self-esteem and interest in a faculty position.

2. Provide a nonthreatening environment, such as inviting a candidate to campus for an informal lunch on a day different from the formal interview. Invite current ethnically diverse faculty to the informal lunch. It is not necessary to have faculty from the same ethnic group since often the number of diverse faculty on campus is small.

3. The composition of the search committee should be well planned. Select ethnically diverse and gender-specific search committee members, including non-tenured faculty. In¬clude faculty that share the same expertise as the candidate. The size of the search committee should be small to increase the comfort of the candidate. Include diverse faculty from other depart¬ments if there are no diverse faculty available in the recruiting department.

4. Preparation for the formal interview is an essential considera¬tion. Provide guidelines and interview questions in advance. Mentor adjunct and part-time faculty in preparation for recruitment to full time. Provide "coaching" assistance with curriculum vitae, mock in¬terviews, and teaching demonstrations to ethnically diverse groups, during workshops such as for nursing organizations, which provide access to a pool of potential faculty.

5. Feedback should be a step of the recruitment process. A candidate should be notified if the process is progressing favorably or if the candidate is not a viable choice as soon as possible by formal and informal means. Often candidates are not given an indication or status of the process. For example, if someone's application is undergoing review or if the review process is on hold for some reason, the candidate should be notified.

**Strategies for Hiring Procedures**

Hiring procedures sensitive to diverse faculty are designed for all candi¬dates as well. Regardless of the candidate's ethnicity, hiring should be based on qualifications. To imply that minorities cannot make it without affirmative action implies less intellectual, leadership, or administrative capability, and that certainly is not true. However, in¬clusion of ethnicity as a hiring consideration is sensitive to diverse faculty candidates. Additionally, experiences other than scholarly activities should be considered as qualifications. Institutions can make a strong commitment to hiring underrepresented minorities through diverse search committees and job descriptions that expand the candidate pool (American Association of State Colleges and Universities, 2006). For example, experiences of a nurse in a lead¬ership role such as a manager or supervisor in a clinical setting may have prepared potential faculty well for supervising nursing students. Nursing departments or schools often use hiring criteria identified by other disci¬plines or human resource units in the college or university. It is essential that nursing faculty be hired using procedures specific to nursing or other health occupations. Just as important is the provision of salary negotiations in line with health occupation practice salaries. When salaries are not com¬parable, incentives can be provided to candidates to encourage the accep¬tance of faculty positions, such as smaller teaching loads, flexible teaching schedules, or release time to pursue scholarly or research activities. Con¬sidering ethnicity as well as degree and experience to determine salary is such an incentive. However, more effective is the provision of a monetary bonus when the candidate is hired. Retention Strategies

Perceived social support, perceived mentorship, and perception of comfort within the university are the strongest predictors of persistence among undergraduate Hispanic students (Gloria, Castellanos, Lopez, & Rosales, 2005). The mentor concept provides a sense of individuality to the retention strategies presented. Aca¬demia has its own unique culture and politics and young or new instructors might need support. Some institutions have assigned a full-time faculty mentor and staff to assist new faculty. The roles of full-time faculty and staff are determined to prevent overlap. Faculty mentors can be prepared for the role in retention by special programs de¬veloped for this purpose. Give monetary bonuses or release time to faculty mentors and staff assigned to orientation of diverse faculty or include in job descriptions, which can be utilized to evaluate performance. As with other strategies, the following additional strategies for retention can be im¬plemented for all new faculty regardless of ethnicity:

1. Develop written orientation programs sensitive to new faculty. In¬clude deans and department heads in the development of orientation programs. Include a checklist to assure all elements of orientation are included. Provide two to three days of formal and structured orienta¬tion.

2. Provide one-to-one orientation to procedures and policies for de¬partment and college, computers and other equipment, campus life and resources, and community resources. Include orientation of physical environment (e.g., bathrooms, kitchen, stairs, and more).

3. Include ongoing orientation through first year for additional expec¬tations. Implement a faculty development plan, which includes guidance on tenure process, teaching effectiveness, grant writing, publications, and campus socialization.

### Strategies for Sensitizing Faculty/Staff to Advantages of Diverse Faculty

It is expected that current faculty and staff will be sensitized by the in¬teraction with the individual faculty candidate as well as the strategies focused on increasing the knowledge about ethnic groups. Once the in¬dividual enters the subsystem of retention, sensitized faculty and staff will impact the retention process. In addition, it is expected that current faculty and staff will become effective participants in the recruitment process as sensitization occurs using the following strategies:

1. Increase culturally diverse media for faculty use in teaching. Imple¬ment a task force consisting of diverse faculty to review, critique, and choose culturally diverse media. Ask faculty to include articles and other references regarding ethnic beliefs and practices into course syllabi.

2. Promote faculty, staff, and student understanding of diversity through workshops and presentations by ethnic speakers, and fac¬ulty, staff, and student meetings. Include workshops that focus on ethnic beliefs and practices of diverse groups, which may affect health care outcomes. Many ethnic nurses have first-hand knowl¬edge of beliefs and practices currently utilized by patients they care for and often can provide insight into how mainstream nurses can intervene with health problems. Continuing education units should be provided for increased participation in workshops and other presentations.

3. Develop a retreat model package, which can be used by other pro¬grams. Implement faculty retreats to increase faculty and staff knowledge about disparity in faculty representation and to iden¬tify advantages of having a diverse faculty and diverse student body. Strategies may include sharing of family experiences with health issues to compare similarities and to identify contrasts. Case studies in which two faculty of dif-ferent ethnicity are asked to solve a nursing problem involving patients from various ethnic groups which can be utilized later in teaching situations.

4. Develop questionnaires to obtain information regarding learning needs, barriers, and problems associated with teaching a diverse population. Often monetary incentives to participants in studies or surveys are useful in gathering large amounts of information. Work¬shops to identify teaching strategies sensitive to the diverse students can be developed from survey results. Focus groups, as well as survey results, can enrich faculty knowledge of diversity and help identify faculty perceptions about diverse students' learning needs.

5. Assign students to clinical preceptors from different ethnic groups to gain understanding of diverse nursing practice influenced by perceptions other than the mainstream population. Many nurses from different ethnic groups have been trained in their native coun¬tries and nursing interventions may be different from what is cur¬rently taught in U.S. nursing schools.

6. Create alliances with ethnic professional health organizations, which may lead to identification of role models, mentors, preceptors, and presenters for classes, seminars, or workshops. These groups often focus on mentoring students and awarding scholarships.

## SUMMARY

The rapid growth of a diverse student population in colleges and univer¬sities has tremendous implications for successful preparation of health care professionals. There is potential to increase the pool of Hispanic and other diverse faculty, which can enhance the academic success of Hispanic students as more enter colleges and universities to become nurses. Matching a diverse student population with diverse ethnic fac¬ulty is one critical approach to addressing recruitment of Hispanics into academia. It is expected that the final outcome will be an increase in diverse faculty and that diverse faculty will in turn participate in different activities to identify potential faculty candi¬dates.

Implementation of any model will put numerous demands on nursing programs and on institutions of learning; however, commitment by the institution will lead to success. The single most important concept in planning and developing re¬cruitment strategies and operationalizing a model or plan is commit¬ment. The strategies presented provide a broad formula on how a teaching insti¬tute can recruit diverse faculty. The first step in operationalizing the ele¬ments of a model or other such initiatives is recognizing the significance of the development of recruitment strategies by ethnically diverse participants who have the expertise, experience, and insight into what will succeed.

# REFERENCES

American Association of Colleges of Nursing. (2008). *Minority Nurse Faculty Scholarship Winners.* In American Association of Colleges of Nursing. Retrieved on July 6, 2012, from http://www.aacn.nche.edu/students/scholarships/minority

American Association of Colleges of Nursing (2010). *Final data from AACN's 2009 survey indicate ninth year of enrollment and admissions increases in entry-level baccalaureate nursing programs.* Retrieved from the American Association of Colleges of Nursing website: http://www.aacn.nche.edu/news/articles/2009/09enrolldata

American Association of Colleges of Nursing (2011, 15 July). *Fact sheet: Enhancing diversity in the nursing workforce.* Retrieved from the American Association of Colleges of Nursing website: http://www.aacn.nche.edu/media-relations/diversityFS.pdf

American Association of Colleges of Nursing. (2012). *Race/ethnicity of students enrolled in generic (entry-level) baccalaureate, master's, and doctoral (research-focused) programs in nursing, 2001-2011.* Retrieved from the American Association of Colleges of Nursing website: http://www.aacn.nche.edu/research-data/EthnicityTbl.pdf

American Association of State Colleges and Universities. (2006, April). *Faculty trends and issues (Vol. 3, No. 4).* Retrieved from the American Association of State Colleges and Universities website: http://www.aascu.org/uploadedFiles/AASCU/Content/Root/PolicyAndAdvocacy/PolicyPublications/FacultyTrends.pdf

Bednash, P. (2003, February 5). *Testimony presentation. Institute of Medicine Committee on Institutional and Policy-level Strategies for Increasing the Diversity of the U.S. Healthcare Workforce.* American Association of Colleges of Nursing. The National Academies, Washington, DC. Retrieved on July 6, 2012 from http://www.aacn.nche.edu/government-affairs/resources/IOM_Test_by_Bednash_2003.pdf

Buchbinder, H. (2007). *Increasing Latino participation in the nursing profession: Best practices at California nursing programs.* Los Angeles, CA: Tomás Rivera Policy Institute.

Calvillo, E. R. (1996). *Recruiting Hispanic nursing faculty.* In S. Torres (Ed.), Hispanic voices: Hispanic health educators speak out. New York, NY: National League for Nursing Press.

Chapa, J., & De La Rosa, B. (2006). The problematic pipeline: Demographic trends and Latino participation in graduate science, technology, engineering, and mathematics programs. *Journal of Hispanic Higher Education, 5*(3), 203-221.

Davidhizar, R., & Shearer, R. (2005).*When your nursing student is culturally diverse.* The Health Care Manager, 24(4), 356-363.

Gloria, A. M., Castellanos, J., Lopez, A. G., & Rosales, R. (2005). An examination of academic nonpersistence decisions of Latino undergraduates. *Hispanic Journal of Behavioral Sciences, 27*(2), 202-223.

Long, B. T., & Kurlaender, M. (2009). Do community colleges provide a viable pathway to a baccalaureate? *Educational Evaluation and Policy Analysis, 31*(1), 30-53.

National League for Nursing. (2010). *NLN nurse educator shortage fact sheet.* Retrieved from the National League for Nursing website: http://www.nln.org/governmentaffairs/pdf/nursefacultyshortage.pdf

Pacquiao, D. (2007). The relationship between cultural competence education and increasing diversity in nursing schools and practice settings. *Journal of Transcultural Nursing, 18*(1), 28S-37S.

Peragallo, N. (2003, November). *Increasing diversity in the nursing workforce: The Hispanic challenge.* (Third Report to the Secretary of Health and Human Services and the Congress). Washington, DC: Bureau of Health Professions, Health Resources and Services Administration.

Pew Hispanic Center. (2009). *Between two worlds: How young Latinos come of age in America.* Washington, DC: Author.

Sullivan Commission on Diversity in the Healthcare Workforce. (2004). *Missing persons: Minorities in the health professions: A report of the Sullivan Commission on Diversity in the Workforce.* Washington, DC: Author.

Taxis, J. C. (2006). Fostering academic success of Mexican Americans in a BSN program: An educational imperative. *International Journal of Nursing Education Scholarship, 3*(1), 1-14.

U.S. Census Bureau. (2011, March). *Overview of Race and Hispanic Origin: 2010.* Retrieved from http://www.census.gov/prod/cen2010/briefs/c2010br-02.pdf

U.S. Census Bureau. (2011, August 26). *Profile America Facts for Features: Hispanic Heritage Month 2011: Sept 15 – Oct 15.* Retrieved from http://www.census.gov/newsroom/releases/archives/facts_for_features_special_editions/cb11-ff18.html

U.S. Department of Health and Human Services. (2010, March). *The registered nurse population.* Initial findings from the 2008 National Sample Survey of Registered Nurses. Washington, DC: Health Resources and Services Administration.

U.S. Department of Health and Human Services. Office of Minority Health. (2008, July 8). *Cultural competency.* In Initiatives. Retrieved on July 6, 2011, from http://minorityhealth.hhs.gov/templates/browse.aspx?lvl=2&lvlID=14

Valverde, M. R., & Rodriquez, R. C. (2002). Increasing Mexican American doctoral degrees: The role of institutions in higher education. *Journal of Hispanic Higher Education, 1*(1), 51-58.

Villarruel, A. M., Canales, M., & Torres, S. (2001). Bridges and barriers: Educational mobility of Hispanic nurses. *Journal of Nursing Education, 40*(6), 245-251.

Wilson, V. W., Andrews, M., & Leners, D. W. (2006). Mentoring as a strategy for retaining racial and ethnically diverse students in nursing programs. *The Journal of Multicultural Nursing & Health, 12*(3), 17-23.

# CHAPTER 6

## JUNTOS PODEMOS (TOGETHER WE CAN): STUDENT-LED MENTORING - A KEY INGREDIENT TO INCREASING THE HISPANIC WORKFORCE IN NURSING

*Norma Martínez Rogers, PhD, RN, FAAN*
*Adelita G. Cantu, PhD, RN*
*Theresa Villarreal, MSN, RN, ACNS-BC*
*Stephanie Acosta*

The growing health disparity gap between minority and majority populations continues to widen in the United States and mirrors the gap between majority and racial and ethnic minority populations in the health professions workforce (Institute of Medicine [IOM], 2002). In the face of growing population diversity in the United States, the lack of minority health professionals has dire consequences for the nation's health (Gardner, 2005). The recent IOM report on the Future of Nursing (2011) charged schools of nursing with improving their educational systems to allow for the seamless progression of nursing students to achieve higher levels of education and training so that they can have a meaningful impact on decreasing health disparities. This chapter describes one school's development and implementation of a student-led mentorship program. This program has been used to successfully recruit, retain, and graduate baccalaureate-prepared Hispanics into the nursing workforce, as well as provided opportunities and resources to seek higher levels of education and training.

## JUNTOS PODEMOS (TOGETHER WE CAN)

Building on the importance of the mentorship process to facilitate success among Hispanic nursing students, a mentoring program called Juntos Podemos (Together We Can) (Cantu & Rogers, 2007) was implemented at the University of Texas Health Science Center at San Antonio, School of Nursing (UTHSCSA-SON). This project was built on the concept of Comadres/Compadres, which in Spanish means friend/pal/confidant. The concept expresses a closeness the significance and depth of which can only be understood by those in the relationship. This relationship provides a means to network; share information about education, culture, and resources; and engage in discussions from the trivial to the significant. It gives one a sense of community and belonging regardless of what is going on in one's life.

The goal of Juntos Podemos is to identify and address the unique needs of Hispanic students by providing a community-based, peer mentoring program that develops interpersonal, organizational, and leadership skills. Juntos Podemos was initiated because of the paucity of Hispanic professional nurses in San Antonio and Texas and the need of UTHSCSA-SON to increase their rate of Hispanic students who graduated from the program. The mottoes of Juntos Podemos are "to strive for excellence" and "in order to receive one must give." Juntos Podemos includes the following four components: (a) service, (b) selection, (c) impact, and (d) evaluation that enable the participants to define the program, implement, and examine its effectiveness.

From the beginning, Juntos Podemos was designed to be a student-led mentoring program. Utilizing the Hispanic tradition of a comadre/compadre relationship, the program is designed to build a continuum of caring. The program matches a lower-level student with a student mentor who is at the next higher level semester (e.g., first-year student with second-year student). Mentors are required to be academically successful in all nursing courses, possess a multicultural awareness, express a willingness to grow, and demonstrate effective interpersonal communication skills.

The mentor-protégé relationship continues as both students progress through the nursing program. One important reason for this process is that mentors, by tutoring their protégés, review content in courses from a previous semester. This allows mentors to more clearly understand how these concepts build upon each other. Consequently, senior students are better prepared for their state board examination because of their constant review of course content with their protégés.

At the beginning of each semester Hispanic faculty advisors involved with the project conduct a one-day intensive training workshop for students who want to join Juntos Podemos. The following four questions frame the discussion: (a) What is mentoring? (b) What is a protégé? (c) What works? and (d) Why does it work? We discuss what it means to be a mentor, focusing on the responsibilities of providing individualized strategies, being available to the protégé for support, and facilitating their development. Similarly the responsibilities of the protégé, which include being available to work with the mentor and the importance of open communication, are also discussed.

The faculty advisors also developed an introductory kit, including an orientation manual for the protégés and mentors, which assists mentors in developing their relationship with students and tracking a student's progress. Based on the premise that there is a strong relationship between faculty involvement and the academic success of nursing students (Alicea-Planas, 2009), the two faculty advisors maintain direct communication through face-to-face and email communication with the mentors and protégés.

During this training workshop, the critical process of matching mentors and protégés is initiated. According to Wroten and Waite (2009) and Robinson and Niemer (2010), important variables for mentor-protégé matching are cultural perspectives, personality style, positive attitudes, and compatibility of professional outlook and goals. To ensure optimal matching, a questionnaire is distributed to the mentors and protégés and responses are used to help faculty advisors match mentors and protégés with similar personalities and learning styles.

It is inevitable that sometimes the mentor-protégé match does not work due to differences in schedules, perspectives, and expectations. For example, a protégé may be self-conscious about independently seeking assistance, while the mentor may have no trouble seeking assistance when needed. The mentor may assume the protégé will come to her or him whenever assistance is needed and because the protégé is reluctant to ask, she or he may not receive the assistance needed to be successful. Such situations are brought to the attention of the faculty advisors and efforts are made to resolve issues; however, reassignment of the mentor or the protégé may occur.

Another example of a mismatch can occur when the protégé or mentor does not have the same racial or ethnic background. Faculty advisors use the opportunity as a teaching moment to discuss how differences not only impact the mentoring relationship but also interprofessional and nurse-patient relationships. Consequently, the protégés who participate in Juntos Podemos develop stronger student-to-student and student-to-faculty relationships.

Protégés also learn to use their expanding support systems to achieve academic goals in a less stressful manner. Mentors enhance their interpersonal, organizational, and leadership skills, while simultaneously earning some financial support. One of the lessons learned from this experience based on comments from past Juntos Podemos members is that the interpersonal and networking skills learned in the program have assisted them in their work settings.

Another component of Juntos Podemos is the development of student profiles by faculty advisors. These profiles include identification of strengths, learning needs, and expressed student concerns. Prescriptive Performance Plans (PPP) are developed for and with the protégés and used to improve study habits and lifestyles choices to maximize their potential. Mentors use the PPPs to monitor and evaluate progress. At each focus group/interview, the mentors and protégés discuss any personal issues impacting their lives as students. The issues are disclosed spontaneously and voluntarily. The process reflects honesty, respect, and confidentiality, and provides individual validation.

### Program Enhancements Due to Consistent Evaluation

We use continuous process improvement methods to consistently evaluate the process and outcomes of Juntos Podemos. Monitored outcomes include the number of students who are and have been academically successful in the nursing program and the number of first semester students who complete the nursing program. Process criteria include participation in required (minimum of eight per semester) face-to-face or email meetings with mentors and protégés or mentors and faculty advisors. Methods of evaluation include formal assessments by the student, mentor, and faculty, as well as informal inputs, such as personal observation, reflective journaling, and both individual and group discussions. An important source of feedback is Family Night, when mentors and protégés share how the program impacts their lives.

A change in the Juntos Podemos program based on students' recommendations, and consistent with the IOM Future of Nursing (2011) recommendation to support higher levels of education and be life-long learners, was to provide students an opportunity to engage in graduate nursing studies. Thus elective courses were offered to prepare students to become a research or teaching scholar. Research scholars were paired with a faculty member conducting research on Hispanic health disparities; teaching scholars were paired with a faculty member to assist with integrating cultural competence content or to assist with providing course content reviews. In addition, a leadership seminar series was developed for those students who were not interested in being a research or teaching scholar.

During process evaluation of Juntos Podemos, we discovered that many students experienced personal and family crises that impacted their studies and grades. Thus, we added a master's level social worker to the program to provide social and emotional support for students, including through brief therapy. In addition, the social worker conducts programs for students related to balancing family, school, and work; self-growth activities; and stress management techniques.

## Impact and Lessons Learned

The impact of Juntos Podemos is evident on academic achievement, performance improvement, retention, and graduation rates. Juntos Podemos has been in existence for 10 years, and since 2004 approximately 2,982 students, predominantly Hispanic, have participated in the program. Ninety-eight percent of the students in Juntos Podemos have been academically successful each semester while in the program. In the past three and a half years, 100 percent of nursing school graduates who have been involved in Juntos Podemos passed the NCLEX on their first attempt. In the past five years, 96 of the 219 fourth semester students in Juntos Podemos have enrolled in graduate school. Finally, past ambassadors of the school of nursing have been mentors in the Juntos Podemos project. In addition to the program, student characteristics such as possessing a strong sense of self, academic interest, and the support of family and/or significant others, contribute greatly to student success. The personal impact of Juntos Podemos can be heard in the voices of a student (see Box 7-1) and alumni (see Box 7-2) who participated in the program.

In addition, Juntos Podemos has helped to create an atmosphere at UTHSCSA-SON that diversity is valued and appreciated. Indeed, Juntos Podemos has helped to create and foster an atmosphere of a caring community and demonstrated that all students at UTHSCSA-SON play a part in everyone's success. Our goal is that this community of caring will be sustainable and continue as the students become nurses and work within collaborative teams. Building and sustaining a community of caring is essential to help graduates redesign health care in their organizations and be leaders in providing patient-centered care.

In conclusion, the peer/mentoring relationship is based on honesty, a strong belief in each other's worth, and the development of collaborative survival skills in the educational process. Participants in Juntos Podemos typically grow beyond the mentor/protégé roles and develop long-term friendships. This is consistent with Robinson and Niemer (2010), who reported that peer support among students was a benefit of the peer mentoring process. Juntos Podemos embraces the Hispanic value of familia y comadres in all aspects of student, peer, and faculty relationships. Juntos Podemos demonstrates that building scholarly and supportive relationships is critical in ensuring educational and personal growth and success.

### Box 6-1  Juntos Podemos – Reflections of a Student

I am a third semester student at the school of nursing and like a majority of the Hispanic population in San Antonio, I was an inner city student. After I graduated from high school in 2003, I started school at a community college where I soon learned how ill-prepared I was to be a successful college student. Nothing went according to plan, primarily because I lacked having a plan. My academics were not my priority. I can recall growing up in a culture that never stressed the importance of obtaining a college education; instead we were bombarded with the infamous D.A.R.E slogan "just say no." My perspective of college was that it was what people who could afford it did after they graduated. I made the decision to attend college during my senior year of high school when I was convinced that it would be affordable because the government would provide tuition assistance.

While other students had been working towards their dreams their entire lives, I was advised that college was a possibility in my future, but never was prepared to be capable of accomplishing what would be expected of me. I had no direction and no one to help guide me along the way. Needless to say, my first attempt in college was unsuccessful. Within less than a year, my GPA fell below a 2.0, which revoked my eligibility to receive financial aid, as well as to continue school. As a result, I was placed on academic suspension and forced to sit out a year before I would become eligible to re-enroll. It was that year that changed my life forever. One year quickly became three years, increasing the likelihood that I would not return to complete my education. My lack of success was in its own way related to my employment, but more so because I quickly became accustomed to accumulating my own income.

In search of a better wage, I quickly changed from one job to another, was in a relationship, moved out, and became a mother a year later. My struggles as a single mother became my fuel and motivation, redirecting me to complete my education. It was my second attempt at the community college that was both the longest and most difficult. I had to undo all the damage I had done to my academic record to prove to both myself and the institution to which I would be applying what I could do.

After completing my associate's degree in science, I was accepted into the UTHSCSA School of Nursing Traditional Baccalaureate program where my new journey would begin. My first semester was one of uncertainty until I was introduced to Juntos Podemos, and joining was the best decision I have made since returning to school. Juntos Podemos continues to give me all the support I need as a new student (and so much more) trying to complete a professional program. The faculty has helped me transition and adapt successfully to the new teaching and testing styles that I have been expected to successfully complete to progress within the program. Most importantly, Juntos Podemos has welcomed me and helped me feel like I belong; they are like family. Following completion of my first semester, I was so grateful that I wanted to contribute to the organization and what it stands for because I learned that alone, completing the program is possible, but can be more difficult. However, as a family, "Together we can" achieve so much more. There will never be any words to describe how grateful I am for meeting such an inspirational group of Juntos Podemos professors who stand by their students and believe in them throughout their journey.

### Box 6-2  Juntos Podemos – Reflections of an Alumnus

Being born to a 13-year old, unwed mother and living in an underserved, undereducated inner city brought many challenges. I was fortunate that my mother encouraged me to gain an education. I graduated at the age of 17 and began college. At the time I was in school, my mother was as well, to "better herself and our lives." She graduated from an associate's degree nursing program.

My early college experience involved being a work-study student in the local community college. My greatest experience was being exposed to the library. I took advantage of the office of admissions where I was assessed as to which areas of study were best for me. This led me to an associate's degree in applied science in nursing, and to a degree in mental health technology. The practica I encountered were important to my own development, as I was a very young college student. My initial reaction to becoming a nurse was one of great excitement and fear, as I was looking for a place to belong and also receive guidance.

As a Hispanic student, I soon realized that my success would depend greatly on the support systems that would be offered to me, which I would accept. During orientation and classes, I always looked for the familiar faces and Spanish surnames to achieve that sense of connectedness. I was looking for my likeness reflected in the faculty, but I did not find it.

**Box 6-2  Juntos Podemos – Reflections of an Alumnus - con't.**

After completing my first semester in the associate's degree nursing program, I began to work in the hospitals. As a nurse extern, I applied my skills in shift work. The feel of the work, the smell of the inner city hospital, and the sounds of technology enchanted me. Soon a new hospital and a new title as a charge nurse found me again as a reluctant leader who recognized the need for more education. The decision to go back to school was harder this time, as I had to make many sacrifices, especially economically and interpersonally. I was also not in a supportive relationship.

When I entered nursing school as a baccalaureate student, there was one program that reached out to me and that was Juntos Podemos. At that point in my life, I was a quiet, reserved student who aspired to become a nursing leader. The leadership development that I wanted and received can be directly linked to the mentorship and guidance received from Juntos Podemos. A connection was formed that still exists to this day, some nine years later. As part of the Juntos Podemos program, I was assigned a mentor who became a friend and confidant with a shared goal of success. My interactions with faculty and peers increased, and I began to transition from a reluctant leader to a confident leader. I discovered I had a voice that had not existed before despite having been a registered nurse for several years.

Throughout the nursing program, the Juntos Podemos mentors and faculty advisors encouraged me to seek a higher level of educational preparedness. "Go on to graduate school" was the charge put forth by the program director. This was a directive that could not have been possible the year before I became a member of Juntos Podemos. I enrolled in graduate school the next semester after graduating with a high degree of academic success, which occurs with many students in Juntos Podemos. Interestingly many mentors and protégés had become classmates and study partners in graduate school. These continued relationships were a testament to successful matching of mentors and protégés.

The Juntos Podemos program created for me a strong sense of belonging, a community of support that continued post-graduate school. This made it considerably easier to transition back into academia as a junior faculty member at the same institution. The values of mentorship and student support continue to be a part of how I view my role as a Hispanic junior faculty member and a faculty advisor for Juntos Podemos.

## References

Alicea-Planas, J. (2009). Hispanic nursing students' journey to success: A metasynthesis. *Journal of Nursing Education, 48*(9), 504-513.

Cantu, A. G., & Rogers, N. M. (2007). Creating a mentoring and community culture in nursing. *Hispanic Health Care International, 5*(3), 124-127.

Gardner, J. D. (2005). A successful minority retention project. *Journal of Nursing Education, 44*(12), 566-568.

Institute of Medicine. (2002). *Unequal treatment: Confronting racial and ethnic disparities in health care.* Washington, DC: The National Academies Press.

Institute of Medicine. (2011). *The future of nursing: Leading change, advancing health.* Washington, DC: The National Academies Press.

Robinson, E., & Neimer, L. (2010). A peer mentor tutor program for academic success in nursing. *Nursing Education Perspectives,* (31)5, 286-289.

Wroten, S. J., & Waite, R. (2009). A call to action: Mentoring within the nursing profession — a wonderful gift to give and share. *ABNF Journal, 20*(4), 106-108.

# CHAPTER 7

## DOCTORAL STUDIES IN NURSING IN MEXICO: THE IMPACT OF GLOBALIZATION

*Bertha Cecilia Salazar-González, PhD, RN, MA, BSN*
*Raquel Alicia Benavides-Torres, PhD, MCE, BSN*
*Esther C. Gallegos, PhD, RN, MBA, BSN*

One of the key recommendations of the Institute of Medicine's Future of Nursing Report (2011) is to double the number of nurses with doctorates by the year 2020. Supporting this recommendation is the realization that expansion of nursing science is essential to providing better patient care, improving health, and evaluating outcomes. In Mexico, while values about research and doctoral education are similar, the development of nursing scientists is in its infancy. The purpose of this chapter is to describe the process of developing and implementing the first doctoral program in nursing offered in Mexico. An overview of graduate education and the position of nursing within higher education will be reviewed. The process followed in planning and conducting the program offered by the Universidad Autónoma de Nuevo León (UANL) is further described, concluding with some considerations on the future of the program in the context of the globalization of higher education.

## GRADUATE EDUCATION IN MEXICO

A country's development is directly linked to the educational attainment of its people. In 2011, Mexico's basic educational level was extended from nine to 12 years of education (Secretaría de Gobernación, 2011). Access to and quality of basic education are foundational to undergraduate and graduate university education. According to the population census of 2010, of the children and youth (six to 14 years) who should attend elementary and middle education, 94.7 percent were enrolled in school. Of youth between 15 and 24 years, only 40.4 percent completed college (Instituto Nacional de Geografía e Informatica, 2010). The segment of the population with access to graduate studies in the country is much lower. Data from 2008-2009 show that nationwide enrollment in master's programs was 166,986 students, while in doctoral programs the enrollment was only 18,530 (Asociación Nacional de Universidades e Instituciones de Educación Superior, 2011).

Doctoral education is a critical component in ensuring the human capital needed to advance knowledge and to create technology required to produce goods and services to address the needs of the country. The development of human capital reduces dependence on foreign technology and more readily fosters global collaborative relationships needed to tackle common problems. Likewise, doctoral graduates are the ideal agents to efficiently and effectively position the country in a globalized market, a characteristic of our modern economy. Globalization is a phenomenon that transcends all dimensions of human life, particularly education. Globalization compels us to think about an equivalent basic education to facilitate effective performance of graduates in any setting. Likewise, globalization puts extreme pressure on the need to increase the number of graduate students trained (Chan, 2008).

It is also important to point out the effect of globalization on health, since decisions to create new graduate programs should be consistent with the interaction between health and globalization. However, it is noteworthy that while health is a worldwide priority, distal determinants of health, such as the lack of fuel and food, climate change, and the financial crisis, often remain as underlying issues affecting health (World Health Organization, 2012). Thus, it is necessary to educate professionals capable of addressing health and developing policies that will affect health at all levels (Kupfer, 2011).

In this regard, during the last two presidential terms, the government of Mexico has taken steps to promote graduate studies within and outside the country. Strategies have included offering scholarships to outstanding students in various disciplines and strengthening national institutions of higher education to offer quality graduate programs. The Science, Technology and Innovation Program (Gobierno de Nuevo León, 2012) highlights the co-responsibility of universities and institutions of higher education in promoting research and innovation to support and strengthen economic development in Mexico. In addition to student and institutional support, efforts are also directed to substantially develop the faculty, so they can extend their efforts and expertise beyond teaching, to focus on research, innovation, and the creation of technology. It is believed that these combined efforts and investment in education will in turn lead to improved living standards.

Considering globalization in the development of human resources, there are aspects such as communication, technology transfer, knowledge of a second language, and other factors that directly or indirectly affect the development of doctoral educational programs. For example, a direct factor impacting quality doctoral education programs are institutional agreements to facilitate student exchange; indirect factors are those related to the country's economy, which facilitate the acquisition of resources for conducting academic programs. In the following section, we describe how these factors influenced the development of the first doctoral program in nursing in Mexico.

## THE DOCTORAL PROGRAM IN NURSING SCIENCE

Since 1970, when the first nursing baccalaureate course was developed, nursing in Mexico has been a university program. Since that time, academic programs, students, and faculty members have been involved in the changes promoted by the government through state universities, the Sub-Ministry of Higher Education, and the National Council of Science and Technology (CONACYT). Nursing has also advanced substantial changes in academia and research through its own associations such as the Mexican Federation of Colleges and Schools of Nursing (FEMAFEE) and more recently by groups that accredit and certify institutions and professionals in the field. Unfortunately, nursing faces difficulty in leading and implementing changes that allow substantial advancements to improve community health.

Undergraduate and graduate nursing programs are primarily offered at state universities and supported primarily by federal funds. This support results in low tuition costs for students and provides access to higher education opportunities. The ability of universities to shift their current educational model to focus on research and innovation is hindered by the lack of financial resources available to support this shift. Competing demands present numerous challenges to move from a teaching-centered model to one that gives research equal importance. The transition requires more professors with graduate degrees and an infrastructure that facilitates research, which until recently has not been the focus of many universities.

Nursing schools are confronted with similar challenges because the majority of schools are part of state universities. Compounding the issue is that there is little recognition and respect for nursing as a scientific discipline and thus skepticism about the ability of nurses to carry out research. It is in this context that the first proposal for a doctoral degree in nursing was presented at one of the top-ranked state universities in Mexico — the Universidad Autónoma de Nuevo León (UANL) and its school of nursing, in the city of Monterrey. The development of a doctoral program in nursing was possible after two professors at the UANL School of Nursing completed their doctoral studies in the United States. These two professors were responsible for the development of the doctoral program with the full support of the university and the school of nursing.

**Planning Process**

There were three different stages in developing a doctoral degree in nursing. The first stage consisted of conducting a needs assessment and the identification of state, federal, and international resources. The second stage focused on the development of a strategic plan that would lead to approval of the doctoral program. The third stage was the development and implementation of an operational plan for the program. Each stage is described.

**Needs assessment.** The first step at UANL was to establish a doctoral committee. The committee was composed of five professors from the Universidad Autónoma de Nuevo León (three from nursing, one from biology, and one from medicine) and three external advisors from international universities (University of Michigan, School of Nursing; Wayne State University, College of Nursing; and Indiana University, College of Nursing). The committee developed plans and oversaw the implementation of the needs assessment. The needs assessment focused on identifying health problems and trends prevalent in the country, projecting unmet health care needs within the current health care system, and identifying opportunities where nursing could lead efforts in addressing those needs. National and local epidemiological and demographic data were reviewed, as well as the current state of higher education. The committee confirmed that nurses had a limited profile in health, education, and research. For example, within the health sector, nursing actions are primarily delegated, so independent actions and their relation to health outcomes were not possible to discern. Within educational settings, nurses as researchers were rare.

A major source of data for the needs assessment came from the perspectives of Mexican nurses. A total of 454 nurses and students from 24 states within Mexico expressed having demands in their jobs that exceeded the training they received. Nurses indicated that doctoral studies in nursing were essential for development of the discipline (46 percent), a basic requirement for improving the population's health care (38 percent), and necessary for clarifying the social relevance of the profession. Similarly, nurses reported that doctoral education was the best resource for defining, extending, and innovating nursing practice (79 percent); evaluating interventions (41 percent); advancing professionalization (39 percent); and for identifying issues of interest for the profession (19 percent).

An additional component of the needs assessment was to understand the characteristics of the potential applicants to the doctoral program. Thus, we analyzed the 33 nursing degree programs and 11 master's programs offered by university schools of nursing in Mexico. Among baccalaureate programs, we found a heterogeneous number of courses or subjects (24-64), highly medicalized content (e. g., medical-surgical, pediatrics, obstetrics, internal medicine, and psychiatry) with varying foci on direct care, nursing procedures (fundamentals of nursing), management (finances), administration (supervision and nursing administration), teaching, and research. An assessment of program objectives revealed the limited scope and complexity of the programs. We analyzed both master's in nursing programs, as well as those offered outside the discipline. The focus of the majority of master's nursing programs was on functional roles (e.g., administration and teaching), as opposed to clinical specialty or research. Few master's' nursing programs, however, were research-oriented and required the development of a thesis.

An assessment of resources was conducted by examining the infrastructure within UANL, the process for the development of doctoral degrees in the country, and the advancement of the nursing discipline in developed countries. Since the 1990s, UANL has supported the policy of creating doctoral programs in schools that have sufficient infrastructure to offer a program at the doctoral level. The school of nursing had both a solid infrastructure and a national reputation of excellence. The school of nursing at UANL at that time had offered the nursing baccalaureate degree for over 40 years and a master's degree for over 30 years. Moreover, during the last 10 years, the master's program, in part because of the distance education capacity, was an important resource for training nursing professors throughout the country. Because of these factors, the proposal received extensive support from the university president's office, including providing the resources necessary for the planning phase.

As part of the needs assessment, doctoral programs offered by UANL and other universities in the country and internationally were analyzed and compared. This analysis was necessary to develop a program that met national and professional standards and was consistent with curricular approaches in doctoral education in both related and unrelated disciplines. The assessment of international programs focused on four of the best doctoral programs in nursing — one in the United States, one in Canada, and two from Brazil. In this part of the process, the growth and development of these academic programs was assessed. Site visits and interactions with colleagues from other countries also served to initiate contacts that would later result in cooperative agreements. The review of doctoral programs within and outside of the discipline affirmed the importance of the following: (a) a research-focused versus teaching-focused doctoral program, and (b) a solid infrastructure for research as a component of doctoral education.

**Strategic planning.** Based on the needs assessment, the second step in our process was to develop a strategic plan for the doctorate in nursing program at UANL. This part of the process involved developing strategies to strengthen the substantive areas within the school of nursing to increase the probability of developing a program of excellence in doctoral studies. Specific areas that were identified included: (a) strengthening the research capacity of master's-prepared professors, and (b) developing and supporting programs of research. To address these areas, we conducted a series of faculty workshops on thesis advising, the use of biomarkers in research, and instrumentation. In addition, we examined the various research projects both completed and in progress in the school. We sought an inclusive theme from which research could be developed and, importantly, would serve as a basis for doctoral education. We initially defined our programs of research as Prevention and Reduction of Risk Factors in Chronic Disease and Exercise as a Nursing Intervention.

A strategic initiative, combined with the previous one, was the decision to educate Mexican faculty in PhD programs abroad. This was a valuable strategy to ensure we would have additional resources at UANL to sustain doctoral education. We recruited interested students who were fluent in English, had a strong statistical base of training, and who had a master's of science in nursing. While this was an important strategy, it is not one we have been able to sustain because funding for studying abroad is scarce.

**Development and implementation.** The approach to curriculum development of the doctorate in nursing was consistent with the regulatory framework of the UANL for designing doctorates. We also enlisted the support of three academics with extensive experience in doctoral education at Indiana University, the University of Michigan, and Wayne State University. Colleagues from these institutions offered their time and expertise to discuss with the planning team critical aspects and program elements necessary for doctoral education in nursing. With this basis, the doctorate in nursing sciences was established requiring a master's degree in the discipline or related field to be admitted. Discussions with external consultants clarified substantive issues and helped to guide decisions about appropriate models of education, as well as specific content.

Some of the guiding principles for program development included the following:

1. The ultimate goal of generating and applying knowledge is to improve the health care of the population.

2. The development of knowledge for the discipline of nursing must be linked to the epidemiological and demographic profiles of the country.

3. The disciplinary knowledge of nursing can guide the development of basic and clinical science, but it is important to consider the knowledge generated in other disciplinary and geographical contexts (universal knowledge).

4. The research problems are grounded in nursing practice.

In addition, advisors confirmed the need for a sufficiently developed infrastructure to be in place before accepting students. Critical components of that infrastructure included existing and robust programs of research and professors prepared to conduct research at the doctoral level. Throughout this process, continued communication and interaction with university graduate authorities was maintained. After a year and a half of uninterrupted work on the project, the program was approved by the University Council.

The doctoral program in nursing had the following characteristics:

*Purpose of the Program.* To train scientists and intellectuals capable of creating and conducting original research and creative work independently to advance nursing knowledge.

*Graduate Profile.* The graduate will be able to do the following: (a) systematically advance knowledge relevant to the nursing profession's goal of promoting overall health and reducing the risk of illness and complications in individuals, groups, and society in general and, (b) exert and provide leadership in research, health and social services systems, and human resources training.

*Curriculum.* The design of the curriculum was based on two basic concepts — health promotion and risk reduction. Both concepts are fundamental to improving the health and welfare of the Mexican population and reducing individual and environmental factors that threaten human health. Potential study phenomena were identified from these two constructs. From the perspective of health promotion, study phenomena include the determinants of health related to human biology, the environment, lifestyle, and the organization of health services. The perspective of prevention and risk reduction included phenomena related to reducing risk factors, protection, early detection, treatment, rehabilitation, and prevention of relapse within population groups or in specific social or health conditions.

Under this framework, four areas or integrating components of the discipline of nursing were identified:

*Theoretical.* Relevant models and theories of nursing, health promotion, prevention and risk approach, and psychosocial theories.

*Substantive.* Essential nursing knowledge.

*Methodological.* Advanced qualitative and quantitative research methods.

*Public Policy.* Concepts and theories that enable formulation and evaluation of social and health policies.

*Cognate.* Interdisciplinary perspectives relevant to specific phenomena and related methodological approaches.

Considering these areas and potential candidates admitted to the program, we developed the curriculum (Facultad de Enfermería, UANL, 2001).

**Implementation.** The curriculum development process culminated in approval by the Honorable University Council (September 2001). The approval took into consideration not only the curriculum design, but also the existence of an infrastructure to guarantee success of the program. We proposed and developed admission criteria and a selection process, a student handbook which included substantive program information from admission through graduation, and performance standards to support program operation. We also designed a curriculum evaluation scheme comprised of outcome and process indicators consistent with quality standards set by the National Council of Science and Technology (CONACYT).

A key part in the program preparation process was the availability of research faculty to support program development. Initially, the most effective way to attain and develop this human resource was through collaborations with research-intensive universities and well established doctoral programs. Thus, exchange and collaborative agreements were established with five universities in the United States and one in Brazil. Short-term collaboration involved obtaining adjunct status for three professors. These faculty gave seminars and served as dissertation advisors and committee members. In addition, five faculty members served as research mentors during students' residence in research in their respective countries.

One of the most difficult aspects in beginning the doctoral program at UANL was the need to develop and conduct externally funded research. Funded research implies that the research is of high quality, significant in its scope, and deemed important to advance science. Through a personal contact with a Mexican-American researcher, we had the opportunity to work collaboratively in a National Institute for Nursing Research-funded randomized controlled trial to test the efficacy of a sexual risk reduction intervention for parents and adolescents. The intervention, named ¡Cuidate! or Take Care of Yourself was developed by Dr. Antonia Villarruel at the University of Michigan and tested with U.S. Latino adolescents, and the purpose of the project was to test it with Mexican adolescents (2001-2008).

The implementation of this research in Monterrey provided invaluable training and learning opportunities in conducting all aspects of a randomized trial — from design, to analysis of results, to dissemination, including publications (Gallegos, Villarruel, Loveland-Cherry, Ronis, & Zhou, 2008). Importantly, the opportunity for nursing faculty and students to participate in research was a component that served as a motivating factor to pursue graduate studies (mainly doctoral education). In addition, the impact of this research was not limited to Monterrey. Supplemental funding supported replication of the research to a semi-rural community in the state of Oaxaca. Faculty took a lead role in implementing the study. To date, a UANL nursing professor has continued to build and expand this program of research.

In addition to infrastructure development at UANL, a program to prepare future professors abroad was simultaneously started to develop nurse researchers who could support the UANL doctoral program. This program involved several strategies. First, we identified and recruited potential candidates. We conducted interviews with outstanding undergraduate students who aspired to pursue graduate studies. Once they were selected, we provided institutional support to prepare them as possible candidates for graduate studies abroad. For two years, they worked to advance their English language, communication, and technology skills. They also enrolled in the master's program in Nursing Sciences at UANL. This provided an opportunity for to become involved in existing programs of research and served as a basis for doctoral studies. Importantly, we were able to secure resources from local and federal institutions to support doctoral studies abroad.

Sending students to obtain their PhDs abroad brought other benefits as we were developing our own doctoral program. For example, one of our professors studied and obtained her PhD at the University of Texas at Austin. Her successful completion can in part be attributed to the fact that she had a specific phenomenon of interest (reducing adolescent sexual risk behavior) prior to the start of her doctoral program. As a result, her focus provided the opportunity to take advantage of more targeted courses and related research activities. Just as valuable was the learning experience in another country, which informed our program development, specifically related to prevention approaches, interdisciplinary learning, and strengthening the link of research to practice and policy.

### Barriers and Strategies to Program Development and Implementation

There have been six cohorts of students admitted since the doctorate in nursing sciences started, and by 2011, 12 students have graduated. Eleven Mexican alumni have returned to their home institutions in different states of Mexico, and a Chilean graduate is working in a nursing school in the U.S. One graduate has become the dean of the nursing school of Universidad de Pachuca, Hidalgo; another one is the chief nurse of the health department in the state of Tabasco. Two other graduates are responsible for the research or graduate studies, and one graduate is in charge of the international mobility program. All continue to teach baccalaureate students. One has been accepted as candidate in Mexico's National System of Researchers. Several other graduates have been awarded national research awards.

Since 2010, we have conducted a comprehensive analysis of the program, including evaluations from faculty and students. As a result of the assessment and in the context of other university and federal requirements and available resources (Secretaría de Investigación, Innovación y Posgrado, 2011), we have made changes. These changes align the program with current advances in science and with changes in educational standards and pedagogy.

While we have had many successes in the program, there are several challenges we are seeking to address. A major issue has been the English proficiency of our students and faculty. Despite overall improvements in English proficiency, it remains one of the most challenging barriers that limits the understanding and dissemination of research in publications and presentations and limits exchange with faculty colleagues from other countries. It has further limited the availability of research experiences and residencies to Spanish-speaking countries or Brazil. We have developed a plan to provide opportunities for English intensive courses during the summer in the U.S. or Canada, but financing such opportunities remains a challenge. One successful strategy that we have employed is to invite international researchers as visiting faculty to expose faculty and students to different perspectives in conducting and presenting research.

The most critical area, however, remains the need to develop human capital in research. For many students, finding expertise in certain areas of science (e.g., genetics) is limited. Thus, the depth of knowledge, resources, and support needed to conduct research at the doctoral level is limited. Further, the numbers, availability, and skill of nursing faculty with doctoral training remain scarce. Some recent graduates have not been able to advance their own programs of research and are not qualified to guide students in their dissertations. There are few opportunities for post-doctoral studies and many faculty members are not able to develop a program of research because the expectations and opportunities for research within their institution are not available.

## GLOBALIZATION IN DOCTORAL EDUCATION IN NURSING

In summary, doctoral education in nursing in Mexico is in its infancy, and we have a long road ahead to ensure we make the impact we know we can make in improving the health of the population. While we have much to do, we also recognize we have accomplished a great deal. We were successful in developing and implementing a doctoral program in nursing. We have been successful in graduating several cohorts of students who are well prepared to conduct independent research and lead health policy changes. Importantly, we have raised the stature of nursing through recognition of our program within CONACYT and also acceptance of many of our PhD graduates and faculty as part of the National System of Researchers.

Our long-term goal is to expand our graduates' area of interest beyond nursing, allowing them to make connections with colleagues from other areas and parts of the world. These connections are facilitated by strong collaborations with international colleagues who were a part of our program development from the beginning and who continue to support the research residence of our students. These opportunities expose students to contexts in which they observe the role of expert researchers, participate in interdisciplinary exchanges, learn advanced methodology, and have access to unlimited published research. This experience further provides an opportunity to network with colleagues from other countries and different areas to create collaborative networks to address issues that are common within our discipline and ultimately address issues that benefit communities in our respective countries.

While we share in the same vision for a bold future of nursing, specifically in the area of development of PhDs, our strategies are different. We remain committed to learning and sharing with colleagues across the border to improve the health of our communities.

# REFERENCES

Asociación Nacional de Universidades e Instituciones de Educación Superior. (2011). Población escolar total según nivel educativo [Student population by educational level]. In *Asociación Nacional de Universidades e Institutos de Educación Superior.* Retrieved on July 9, 2011, from http://www.anuies.mx/servicios/e_educacion/docs/web_2008_2009/ GENERAL2009-1.xls

Chan, M. (2008). *Globalización y salud.* Retrieved from World Health Organization website: http://www.who.int/dg/speeches/2008/20081024/es/

Gallegos, E. C. (2001, February 6). P*ropuesta de programa de Doctorado en Ciencias de Enfermería.* [Proposal for a Ph.D. program in Nursing Science]. Secretaría de Programas de Doctorado, Facultad de Enfermería, Universidad Autónoma de Nuevo León.

Gallegos, E.C., Villarruel, A.M., Loveland-Cherry, C., Ronis, D.L., and Zhou, Y. (2008). Intervención para reducir riesgo en conductas sexuales de adolescentes: Un ensayo aleatorizado y controlado [Adolescent sexual behavior risk reduction intervention: a randomized and controlled study]. *Salud Pública de México, 50,* 1-10.

Gobierno de Nuevo León. (2012). Programa estratégico de ciencia, tecnología e innovación: programa especial: plan estatal de desarrollo 2010-2015 [Strategic program for science, technology, and innovation: Special program: state development program 2010-2015]. In *Instituto de Innovación y Transferencia de Tecnología.* Retrieved on July 9, 2012, from http://www.mtycic.com.mx/docs/ped.pdf

Institute of Medicine. (2011). *The future of nursing: Leading change, advancing health.* Washington, DC: The National Academies Press.

Instituto Nacional de Estadística y Geografía (INEGI). (2010). Principales resultados del censo de población y vivienda 2010. [Main results from the population and housing census 2010]. In *INEGI* website. Retrieved April 18, 2012 from : http://www.censo2010. org.mx/

Kupfer, A. (2011). Towards a theoretical framework for the comparative understanding of globalisation, higher education, the labour market and inequality. *Journal of Education and Work, 24*(1-2), 185-208.

Secretaría de Educación Pública. (2011). Articulación de la educación básica (Acuerdo número 592). [Articulation of basic education (Agreement No. 592)]. In *Secretaría de Gobernación* website. Retrieved April 18, 2012 from: http://basica.sep.gob.mx/ reformasecundaria/doc/sustento/Acuerdo_592_completo.pdf

Secretaría de Investigación, Innovación y Posgrado, Universidad Autónoma de Nuevo León. (2011). *Modelo académico de posgrado: Primera actualización* [Post Baccalaureat Academic Model: First Update]. In Universidad Autónoma de Nuevo León. Retrieved on March 12, 2012, from http://www.uanl.mx/sites/default/files/Modelo.Academico.posgrado.pdf

World Health Organization. (2012). *Globalization and health*. Retrieved from http://www.who.int/trade/glossary/story044/en/index.html

# CHAPTER 8

## REFLECTION: A STUDENT'S PERSPECTIVE ON STUDYING IN LATIN AMERICA

*Carmen Alvarez, PhD, RN, NP-C, CNM*

## LEARNING FROM ABROAD FOR THE FUTURE OF NURSING

Regardless of the profession, international work experience is a priceless opportunity. It affords the development of new perspectives, personal growth, and cultural sensitivity. According to Florence Nightingale (1860), a nurse "ought to study them [his or her patients] till she feels sure that no one else understands them so well." It is not until nurses are willing to understand those in their care that they can provide the best holistic care possible, whether it is at the bedside or in a larger community setting. A benefit of immersion in the life and culture of another country is seeing how and why people live the way they do. It becomes apparent that not all behavior is a choice, but, often, the consequence of economic, social, and political constraints and opportunities. Appreciating the complex influences on health outcomes and human behavior provides an essential perspective from which to derive health care solutions.

For these reasons, international experience is paramount. Unfamiliar situations create a type of discomfort that begs the newcomer to reflect on the self. A stranger must develop communication and other skills to get along with other people no matter how dissimilar they may be. This essay is a reflection on two particular international experiences that I had during my undergraduate education. My intent is to share how these two invaluable experiences enhanced my personal growth, shaped my perspectives about nursing, and influenced my current research trajectory.

## THE MINORITY IN INTERNATIONAL RESEARCH TRAINING PROGRAM (MIRT)

Ethnic and gender disparities in health care are not only apparent in patient outcomes, but also in the health care and the composition of research professionals who contribute to the advancement of health care and health promotion. In an effort to address these disparities, the Fogarty International Center and the National Center for Minority Health and Health Disparities, both part of the National Institutes of Health, funded the MIRT program (Fogarty International Center, 1999). The main objective of the MIRT program is to expose qualified undergraduate students (and some graduate students) to health-oriented international research projects. The trainees become more aware of global health issues but also, hopefully, are inspired to pursue careers in the health, biomedical, or behavioral sciences and continue to explore health challenges of marginalized or underserved groups.

To carry out this mission, faculty from health science departments at universities who have collaborated with organizations outside of the United States volunteer to mentor a trainee on a research project. Although the trainee may identify country and research project preferences, similarity in research interest between the trainee and study is the main factor that is used to match the trainee with a mentor. Since the research project is a collaboration between U.S. and foreign country institutions, the trainee also usually has a mentor from each institution. The program is from 10 to 12 weeks in duration, and at the end of the experience, the student is expected to produce a final research paper and report on their experience in the country.

### My First MIRT Experience

My advisor first introduced me to a MIRT program in the spring of 2002 during my baccalaureate junior year of my nutritional science program at Iowa State University. My research interests in non-communicable chronic diseases matched with research at the Center for Studies of Sensory Impairment, Aging and Metabolism (CeSSIAM) in Guatemala and the University of Alabama at Birmingham School of Public Health. I was assigned to work with an interdisciplinary group of research experts from both institutions, including physicians, nutritionists, and epidemiologists.

One of the many joint research projects included a large cross-sectional study on chronic diseases among indigenous populations. My research topic was "The Prevalence of Obesity in Urban Mayan Women, and Its Relationship with Diabetes and Hypertension." This was my first experience conducting research where I developed my own research question, completed the data analysis, and wrote a paper. Prior to embarking on this experience, I had never even written a literature review and I had one basic 100-level statistics class. Fortunately, as a McNair scholar, I had a mentor who shared with me insights about how to use databases, such as MEDLINE, when looking up research articles. With this arsenal, I felt well equipped to complete my assignment. I was humbled in little time.

MIRT also makes the much-appreciated gesture of sending students in pairs. My travel mate was a pre-med student from Xavier University in Louisiana who was just as "prepared" as I was for doing research and had the extra challenge of not knowing any Spanish. We arrived at a time in the project when data had only been collected on women and still needed to be collected for men. As the focus of the project was on indigenous groups, the study site was a couple hours away from Guatemala City, in Quetzaltenango (better known to the locals as Xela, pronounced Che-la), the second largest city in Guatemala, which has a large population of indigenous persons. We initially spent most of our time in Xela assisting with data collection for the first several weeks and simultaneously going to Spanish school. Since I was fluent in Spanish, I spent the mornings in class for the first couple weeks to brush up on my language skills, and then spent the afternoons in internet cafes collecting research articles for my literature review.

In addition to the research project, the cultural immersion and living with Guatemalan families revealed how environment, lifestyle, language, and being of a "socially less-desirable ethnic group" impacted health. It was interesting to see the how migration from rural to urban areas resulted in a population with higher rates of overweight and obesity and chronic diseases. Prevention was not as simple as just exercising and eating healthy. Here were people who had a recent history of being physically and psychologically abused by the system, were generally poor, and had high illiteracy rates as a result of being prohibited from going to school. Where do you start talking about food "choices" in a population that is struggling to meet their basic needs?

Although I was still very much a novice, the research skills I learned from this experience resulted in a paper that was submitted for publication. The following spring I presented a poster of my research at the Experimental Biology conference in San Diego, California. The other MIRT trainee also completed a paper and presented her project to the CeSSIAM group entirely in Spanish.

## International Nursing Experience with MIRT

Although I was initially on a track to medical school, my experience with MIRT in Guatemala rekindled my interests in community health and holistic health care, and hence, I started to consider nursing as a career. Ironically, on one of my many weekend excursions while in Guatemala — a hike up a volcano — I met a nurse who was on vacation from Colorado. Over the grueling, steep, eight-hour uphill hike, he shared his experience and passion for nursing. Almost a year later, I was enrolled in the BSN-MSN program at the Nell Woodruff Hodgson School of Nursing at Emory University in Atlanta.

Because I learned so much from my Guatemala experience, before I had even completed a semester of nursing school, I started exploring available MIRT programs, now known as the Minority Health and Health Disparities International Research (MHIRT) Program (National Institute on Minority Health and Health Disparities, n.d.). To my surprise, I found a nursing-focused MHIRT opportunity at the University of Illinois at Chicago College of Nursing. Although I was now in nursing school, I was not familiar with nursing research outside a clinical setting. My eagerness to learn more about nursing research, was (and still is) driven by my belief that research is one of the better avenues to address health inequities.

Shortly after notification of my acceptance to the program, I received an e-mail stating that I was assigned to go to Monterrey, Mexico, where I would be working on an HIV prevention project. I initially was not pleased with my assignment; I had been to Mexico many times and Brazil was my first choice. For a brief moment, I thought about declining the offer. However, I am more than grateful that I quickly came to my senses because MHIRT in Mexico led me on what thus far has been an exceptionally rewarding path in nursing research, and it is really just the beginning.

Another MHIRT trainee from the College of Nursing at the University of Illinois in Chicago and I were assigned to the *¡Cuidate!* study (Villarruel, Zhou, Gallegos, & Ronis,

2010), a project that focused on HIV prevention in adolescents through education of both adolescents and their parents. I specifically investigated the parents' comfort discussing sex with their children before and after the intervention. In addition to completing a research project, we also made it a point to explore the health care system, nursing education, and of course, the country.

Although the ¡Cuidate! project was in its final stages, we were able to participate in some very important components of the study. On several occasions, we prepared and assisted with the follow-up sessions, which gave me a new appreciation for what it means to conduct a randomized control trial with follow up on such a large scale. A great deal of meticulous preparation was involved in getting all the research materials together, not to mention the reminders that had to go out to adolescents and their parents. The turnout of return participants was impressive. The way in which the follow-up data collection sessions flowed and the participation of adolescents and parents spoke to the excellent teamwork among the staff and the camaraderie and respect that the staff had with the participants. Those of us in science have read and perhaps encountered mistrust of a community for researchers because of violation of bio-ethical issues. One could safely infer that such participation in the ¡Cuidate! project also reflected how personally rewarded the participants felt by having attended the sessions. In addition, this was also a reflection on the level of trust and confidence that the participants had for the researchers.

We also had the opportunity to observe focus groups with the facilitators of the intervention. All the facilitators discussed how they had been positively impacted by teaching the sessions. Both of these experiences demonstrated how research projects can have subtle yet profound impacts beyond the intended target groups, making the project that much more valuable. I felt as though this participatory approach helped provide the community a sense of ownership for the project and outcome.

**Nursing and Health Care in Mexico**

We were also afforded several opportunities to learn more and gain an understanding about the health care system in Mexico. With the help of the co-principal investigator, we met with nurse-directors at some major hospitals in the city and nurses in the community health sector. We also had a shadowing experience at one of the hospitals. Coming from the U.S., a developed country where health care is not a right, I was impressed by the existing systems geared towards making health care services available to all Mexicans despite the limitations of geographical access to health care services. In the United States, this same issue of making health care available to all is still unresolved, expensive, contentious, and continues to be a hot political campaign matter. Is there something we can learn from our neighbors?

We also learned about the complex nursing education system. Despite differences in our health care systems, we face similar challenges regarding the nursing shortage and nursing education (American Nurses Association, 2011). For example, Mexico also has several entry points into the profession to address workforce demands. These entry points included diploma programs and associate's and BSN programs. The lack of standardization in nursing education has implications for the respectability of the nursing profession among the public and other health care professionals. For example, nurses are not considered "professionals," but "workers." Our visit to the vibrant state of Oaxaca, a southern and rural state, provided yet another interesting perspective about health care and nurses. It was during this time that I was exposed to the frequent clash between the culture of health care and that of the population being served. The demographic profile in Oaxaca is very different from Monterrey, in that the population is largely indigenous, while in Monterrey the population is mostly Ladino (an ethnic group that has both indigenous and European heritage). Nurses in Oaxaca were primarily Ladino. We witnessed several instances of cultural insensitivity by nurses, including blaming patients and disrespecting indigenous traditions, including the use of lay healers and the type of clothing worn.

**Lessons Learned**

The MHIRT programs challenged us to think critically about problems that we recognized and steered us in directions that enabled us to gather and understand the context of increasing obesity or the nursing shortage. This experience definitely helped to broaden my perception of policy and its importance in the advancement of the nursing profession both nationally and internationally. These experiences helped me realize the similarity of health care issues between countries and the opportunities for collaboration. The nursing shortage and issues regarding nursing education are matters not only specific to Mexico but are also relevant here in the U.S. and other countries as well. The care and passion that we put into advocating for our patients should also be applied to transforming the nursing profession so we are equipped to better serve all sectors of populations worldwide.

On a personal note, the experience of having to live in a country in which you are not a native inevitably exposes you to uncomfortable or offensive experiences. Even though I did not have a language barrier in Mexico, as an Afro-Latina I was clearly an outsider and, at times, drew stares that made me uncomfortable. As a person who had done a lot of traveling and considered myself to be culturally competent, this experience challenged me to do more for my patients when I returned to the U.S. Beyond putting my own beliefs aside, I can empathize with the challenges of being away from home.

### The Relevance of my International Experiences to Where I Am Today

When I returned to Emory, I did what I could to stay involved in research and to keep in touch with my mentors; I kept in contact with Dr. Villarruel. Most of my clinical rotations during my master's program were with underserved populations, and the more I worked with this community the more I thought about how research could potentially be of benefit by deciphering solutions to community health problems. I became particularly interested in health behaviors and health promotion. After consultation with all my mentors, I applied to the PhD in nursing program at The University of Michigan School of Nursing, worked with advisor and mentor Dr. Villarruel, and in 2012 successfully completed the program. My research focus is on sexual communication among young adult, heterosexual Latinos in relationships, and the influence of sexual communication on sexual behavior. Although my research is informed by my disciplinary perspective, my international research experiences have helped me to maintain an open mind in approaching the challenge of HIV prevention.

Another benefit of my research experiences abroad are the connections I made. Maintaining contact with faculty in Monterrey, for example, has provided the opportunity for collaboration on a publication, as well as provided me with additional expertise during my dissertation study. Since it is my goal to replicate my current research abroad, my established linkage can hopefully facilitate further collaboration on research projects that will be useful to communities in the United States and Mexico.

## CONCLUSION

Acknowledging the growing demands on the nursing profession, the Institute of Medicine (IOM) (2011) underscored the importance of advancing the nursing profession and discipline. The recommended changes include reforming education to produce nurses not only with "task-based proficiencies" but also dynamic critical thinkers who can navigate the multiple facets of nursing to contribute to quality patient care, in-patient, as well as in the community. Programs such as MHIRT and other service learning opportunities abroad can help contribute to the preparation of nursing scholars and care providers. The lessons learned from my research experiences were invaluable and could never be realized within a typical nursing school curriculum.

Although the MHIRT program is research focused, learning about research is only part of the experience. The awareness developed about global issues, and consequently the context sensitive perspective from which to view public and individual health issues, are additional personal and professional benefits. In general, studying abroad facilitates research collaboration, provides for the development of career networks, and the exposure to a new environment encourages ingenuity. Such experiences are critical for advancing the future of nursing, in which nurses around the globe, through research, education, and practice, can transform health care.

## REFERENCES

American Nurses Association. (2011). *Understanding the nursing shortage and what it means for patients.* Retrieved from http://www.nursingworld.org/ FunctionalMenuCategories/ MediaResources/MediaBackgrounders/Nursing-Shortage-Backgrounder.pdf

Fogarty International Center. (1999). *Minority International Research Training Grants.* RFA No. TW-99-001. Retrieved from http://grants.nih.gov/grants/guide/rfa-files/RFA-TW-99-001.html

Institute of Medicine. (2011). *The future of nursing: Leading change, advancing health.* Washington, DC: The National Academies Press.

National Institute on Minority Health and Health Disparities. (n.d.). Minority health and health disparities international research training program. In *National Institute on Minority health and Health Disparities.* Retrieved on July 10, 2012, from http://www. nimhd.nih.gov/our_programs/mhirt.asp

Nightingale, F. (1860). *Notes on nursing: What it is and what it is not.* Retrieved from the University of Pennsylvania website: http://digital.library.upenn.edu/women/nightingale/ nursing/nursing.html

Villarruel, A. M., Zhou, Y., Gallegos, E. C., & Ronis, D. L. (2010). Examining long-term effects of ¡Cuidate! – a sexual risk reduction program in Mexican youth. *Revista Panamericana de Salud Publica/Pan American Journal of Public Health, 27*(5), 345-351.

# CHAPTER 9
## THE USE OF INNOVATIVE TECHNOLOGIES AS A STRATEGY TO ENSURE HISPANIC NURSING STUDENT SUCCESS

*Laura Gonzalez, PhD, RN, APRN, CNE*
*Jean Giddens, PhD, RN, FAAN*

For the past decade, concerns about the lack of workforce diversity in nursing have been raised because of the impact on quality of health care delivery (Institute of Medicine, 2004; Sullivan Commission on Diversity in the Healthcare Workforce, 2004). Recognizing the need to address this issue, many nursing schools have responded through recruitment and enrollment efforts targeting underrepresented minority students. According to the American Association of Colleges of Nursing (AACN) (2010), the population of students enrolled in baccalaureate nursing programs has become increasingly diverse over the past 10 years – from 17 percent minority enrollment in 2001 to 26.5 percent in 2010. America's nursing workforce is also becoming more diverse. Comparisons made between the 2000 and 2008 nursing workforce survey reveal an increase of 4.3 percent in minority nurses — from 12.5 percent to 16.8 percent (Health Resources and Services Administration [HRSA], 2000, 2010). Although progress has been made when considering percentages of minority groups collectively, increases in Hispanic students enrolled in nursing programs and increases in the number of Hispanic nurses in the workforce lag compared to other minority groups. Enrollment of Hispanic/Latino students increased only 2.5 percent in nursing programs during the last 10 years (AACN) and there has been only a 1.6 percent increase in the nursing workforce since 2000 (HRSA, 2010). According to the latest national workforce survey, only 3.6 percent of the nursing workforce is Hispanic (HRSA, 2010). This is especially concerning considering that Hispanics account for an estimated 16.3 percent of the national population (United States Census Bureau, 2010).

These statistics speak to the need for nursing faculty to create an academic environment that is inviting to Hispanic students. Hispanic Americans comprise the nation's largest minority group and the delivery of culturally competent care by Hispanic nurses can favorably impact the health of the Hispanic population. For this reason, it is in the nation's best interest to ensure the success of Hispanic nursing students. As admissions of Hispanic students increase now and in the future, nurse educators must consider perceptions of the academic environment among Hispanic students and respond with teaching strategies and a learning environment more suited to their learning preferences.

## HISPANIC NURSING STUDENTS AND LEARNING PREFERENCES

There are many known barriers to success among Hispanic nursing students; top among them are non-flexible curricula and the existence of power differentials (Moceri, 2010). Elements such as institutional culture, student resources, and faculty-student interactions must also be considered. The application of teaching strategies that enhance Hispanic student retention and academic success is needed. Pappamihiel and Moreno (2011) recommend the use of culturally responsive teaching — a pedagogy that recognizes the importance of including the students' cultural identity in all aspects of teaching. Hispanics, by nature, are a collective culture, which suggests they value group interaction (Velez-McEvoy, 2010). Thus it is not surprising that many Hispanic learners thrive in collaborative and high-context learning environments (Ibarra, 2001). Group work and collaboration allow for a sense of community building, which tends to be highly valued among Hispanic learners. Furthermore, active engagement tends to create a sense of ownership in the learning process for these learners (Pappamihiel & Moreno). Moceri recommends faculty incorporate learning activities and assignments that encourage cooperation over competition. This is viewed as positive and helpful in ensuring a safe learning environment. According to Moceri, a safe learning environment is a framework wherein the students feel safe to express their opinions and viewpoints; this concept has been shown to result in success in learning.

Giddens (2008) identified the need for nurse educators to embrace alternative models of teaching and innovative strategies to ensure the success of underrepresented nursing students such as Hispanics. Two innovative learning technologies used in nursing education, virtual communities and simulation, are presented in this chapter. These innovative learning technologies link to the high-context learning preferences of many Hispanic students, contribute to a safe learning environment, and ultimately lead to student success.

## Innovative Technologies for Learning

The majority of baccalaureate nursing students today are millennial learners born between 1980 and 2000. For the majority of these students, technology has been a component of their everyday life and the use of technology in educational settings comes naturally. There are several types of technology used in nursing education today, including virtual communities (VC), simulation, blogging, audience response systems (ARS), podcasting, and personal digital assistants (PDAs) to name a few. The use of technology in teaching can increase student engagement because it requires direct student participation. Student-centered, active learning is especially powerful when collaboration is required.

**Virtual communities.** A virtual community (VC) is a web-based application featuring the stories of characters that represent diverse cultures and backgrounds. The story lines of VCs developed for nursing and health sciences education feature health-related issues and issues associated with health care delivery. The VC stories are usually enhanced with medical histories and health records, photos, video clips, and community specific data. The following three virtual communities have been described in the nursing literature: the Neighborhood (Giddens, 2007, 2008), Mirror Lake (Curran, Elfrink, & Mays, 2009) and Stillwell (Walsh, 2011).

A defining characteristic of VCs is context. Faculty develop learning activities that link to the character stories, thereby creating a context for students as they learn about nursing and health care issues. The emphasis for learning is gaining understanding and perspective through the experiences of the community characters and their life situations. When used in this way, VCs capitalize on the "power of context" described by Benner, Sutphen, Leonard, & Day (2010) as a process in which skills are translated to a higher level of thinking. The use of a virtual community as a basis for teaching also facilitates integrative learning, linking clinical situations to the classroom and vice versa. The VC not only provides students with context to enhance learning, but it also enhances student engagement by adding an additional level of complexity and richness.

Another advantage of a VC is the ability to present nursing beyond the context of the acute inpatient care setting. The VC allows students to experience a wide array of health-related events experienced by individuals, including health promotion and wellness, acute non-threatening illness, and the progression of chronic illnesses, including exacerbations. This community-based lens also provides an opportunity to view family and community responses to health-related events.

The VC represents a pedagogical shift from content driven didactic instruction to a learner-centered approach (Kantor, 2010). Because stories unfold over time, VCs foster a forward thinking perspective; in other words, students are encouraged to consider issues and future events, as well as alternative actions. Gonzalez and Fenske (2012) reported success using a VC in small discussion groups with nursing students. The authors created an environment that encouraged discussion, dissension, critical thinking, and the development of clinical judgment by posing questions based on VC characters. Purposeful, context-based discussion provides a basis for knowledge acquisition and application.

***Virtual communities and engagement in nursing education.*** The use of VCs is still relatively new and outcomes associated with use are beginning to emerge. A review of the literature revealed eight published research studies in the nursing literature using virtual communities; all but one study evaluated the Neighborhood (Giddens, 2007, 2008). The first studies were conducted shortly after the development of the initial version of the Neighborhood. In one study of 248 baccalaureate nursing student participants, the students with the greatest perceived benefit for learning included underrepresented minority students and students who expected to receive a course grade below an A (Giddens, Shuster, & Roerigh, 2010). The researchers also reported that the perceived benefit increased over time. In a second study, a qualitative analysis of written responses among a group of 40 nursing students who used the Neighborhood for three semesters revealed two primary themes — emotional connectedness and integration. Emotional connectedness refers to the connection students gained to the characters. Evidence of emotional connection was gained though positive or negative comments about a character. Examples included an expressed concern for a character, expression of empathy, or occasionally frustration or anger at a character. Integration refers to the ability to make connections between character events and content learned in the clinical or classroom setting. Both of these findings are associated with learner engagement (Giddens, Shuster, & Roerigh).

Studies were also conducted at five nursing programs beta-testing the Neighborhood in 2008. Results from these studies showed a significant relationship between frequency of use of the Neighborhood and perceived benefits; that is, students reported increased learning benefit as faculty use increased. Although this study did not directly measure the number of times or ways faculty used the intervention, use was indirectly measured through student report of use (never, a few times, occasionally, often). There was no evidence of a relationship between a student's learning style and preference for using the VC (Fogg, Carlson-Sabelli, Carlson, & Giddens, in press). Additional findings included greater learning engagement in the nursing program reported among minority students compared to white students using the VC (Giddens, Fogg, & Carlson-Sabelli, 2010), and greater cultural awareness among students with greater VC exposure/use compared to students with little to no exposure (Giddens, North, Carlson-Sabelli, Rogers, & Fogg, 2012). In another study, a content analysis approach was used to evaluate the benefits and challenge responses of 281 nursing students using the Neighborhood. Three benefit themes were identified. The first, enlarged view, links to students' greater understanding of factors that impact the health care individuals and families across time and complexity of health problems. A second theme, clarity of concept application, refers to the students' perception that the VC helped them connect information learned in the classroom to real-life situations. The third theme, engagement, is described by the feeling that characters and their situations come to life through stories (Carlson-Sabelli, Giddens, Fogg, & Fiedler, 2011). These themes are very similar to those reported by Shuster, Giddens, and Roerigh (2011).

Walsh and Crumbie (2011) reported similar results based on a focus group of students who used the Stillwell virtual community. Students reported the VC allowed them to relate theory to practice in ways they had never done before; the researchers also reported that students developed an emotional connection with the characters. Finally, in another study (Giddens, Hrabe, Carlson-Sabelli, Fogg, & North, in press), the learning engagement, communication exchanges, quality of instruction, and academic performance among a group of nursing students using the VC on one campus was compared to a group of nursing students on another campus. Both groups were from the same institution and both campuses followed an identical curriculum. Learning engagement and communication exchanges were significantly higher among students using the VC. The two groups were very similar in how they rated the quality of instruction and academic performance.

The common themes that emerged from the body of literature to date include the following: students have higher preferences for the VC and have greater engagement when faculty use the technology effectively in the classroom. This represents, in fact, a dose and efficacy effect. The early evidence from three studies also suggests a preference for learning and/or increased perceived benefits to learning with a VC among minority students. When faculty do not use the VC effectively or frequently, students are less likely to report benefits.

This underscores the need for faculty to be open to teaching benefits using alternative learning applications, such as a VC.

**Simulation.** Simulation is a teaching strategy that has been widely adopted in nursing school curricula over the past decade. According to Velez-McEvoy (2010), simulation represents a friendly education paradigm. When implemented optimally, simulation levels the playing field in favor of the learners through a collaborative approach to learning. Students who participate in simulation benefit from the following four learning approaches: visual, auditory, tactile, and kinesthetic (Jeffries, 2007).

*Types of Simulation Environments.* Simulation relies on the creation of an authentic environment; this authenticity is referred to as fidelity. The simulated environment can be low-fidelity, mid-fidelity, or high-fidelity. Low-fidelity simulation involves the use of static mannequins and task trainers which do not respond physiologically, such as an intravenous arm model for practicing intravenous insertion. Mid-fidelity simulation utilizes mannequins that can be programmed with basic functions, such as the VitalSim™, but these mannequins do not interact with the environment. High-fidelity simulation typically uses a human patient simulator which approximates reality by responding physiologically to certain interventions, such as medication administration, fluid resuscitation, and physical positioning. Fidelity can be further enhanced by paying special attention to the spatial environment and incorporating realistic variables such as call bells, ringing phones, and noxious smells. High-fidelity simulation has been found to improve competencies through purposeful repeated practice (Garrett, MacPhee, & Jackson, 2010).

The two most common simulation approaches are formative and summative evaluative applications. Formative simulation emphasizes learning. It provides an opportunity for students to be evaluated and receive feedback in a non-punitive, non-judgmental environment. This process is utilized with the goal of addressing student deficiencies and providing feedback for improved performance. A benefit of formative simulation is that it allows students an opportunity for group think; in other words, students collaborate on the care of a patient in a safe environment. This is best done in learning groups of approximately four students with one facilitator. Additionally, the assignment of roles and tasks (such as primary nurse and scribe) allows students to focus on their roles and understand the dynamic interplay of the health care team.

The use of simulation in summative evaluation typically refers to a high-stakes simulation evaluation used for program advancement and testing purposes. The National League for Nursing is currently exploring the use of simulation for high-stakes assessment. The project is in its second year and is being led by a panel of nationally recognized experts in the field of simulation. The researchers hope the findings will inform national curriculum decisions on preparation for entry into practice (Rizzolo, Oermann, Jeffries, & Kardong-Edgren, 2011).

***Benefits of Simulation.*** Positive learning outcomes can be achieved by using any of the various levels of simulation. The desired learning outcomes dictate the type of simulation to use. Several benefits to simulation have been documented, such as enhanced critical thinking, self-awareness, and self-efficacy (Ironside & Jeffries, 2010). Another benefit of simulation is that nursing students are allowed to learn in a safe environment, free from serious repercussions and fatal outcomes.

A recent study compared simulation and traditional clinical experiences related to enhancing nursing students' knowledge (Gates, Parr, & Hughen, 2012). The results support the effectiveness of simulation in increasing overall knowledge, and the idea that it may be a viable substitute for clinical experiences. What is most intriguing about the study is that low-performing students may have exhibited a slight boost on exam performance after simulation. The researchers caution that without adequate statistical power, this finding needs to be interpreted cautiously. Despite this caveat, one wonders if the low performers identify with underrepresented minority students such as Hispanics. This information may help to further understand the learning preferences of Hispanic and underrepresented students in general.

Another important benefit of simulation is the ability to standardize learning experiences for all participants. Nursing faculty recognize there are important clinical situations that may not readily become available during the clinical rotation; yet exposure to such experiences is critical to student success. Simulated experiences focusing on such clinical experiences are often referred to as low-volume, high-risk scenarios. These include situations such as post-partum hemorrhage, a blood transfusion reaction, anaphylaxis, shock, or impaired airway, to name a few. During simulated experiences such as these, all students are exposed to the same objectives, same pitfalls, and similar expected learning outcomes.

Debriefing is a very important component of simulation. The debriefing process is sometimes referred to as the after-action review, where students often have that "ah-ha" moment. With guidance from the facilitator, students have an opportunity to crystallize their thinking and come to terms with their ideas relative to the patient they just cared for. Debriefing promotes critical thinking and increases self-confidence, while promoting self-reflection.

When optimally applied, simulation reflects a caring environment, one which allows for analysis of problems and acquisition of skills (Velez-McEvoy, 2010). Among Hispanic nursing students, small group interaction decreases student anxiety and helps them attain basic skills and preparedness for didactic courses. As a word of caution, small group learning, when not approached correctly, can lead to heightened anxiety and cause feelings of intimidation (Micari & Drane, 2011), especially among ethnic minorities and underrepresented students. Faculty need to be cognizant of these issues and ensure a level playing field. It is recommended to pre-brief and explain to the participants the objectives and the concept of "group think." Likewise, it is important to reinforce the idea of a safe environment and to ensure an individual student's performance is confidential. Some faculty prefer to assign students to simulation groups based on prior performance so the overall knowledge of the group is similar, as opposed to having one or two strong students who may dominate the experience. This can lead to a sense of frustration and feelings of inadequacy among the other participants. Evidence suggests when competence threat is eliminated, there is an opportunity for Hispanic and underrepresented students to process information at a deeper level (Micari & Drane).

**Link of Virtual Community and Simulation Use to Hispanic Learners**

There are often incongruities between teaching styles and student learning styles. According to Flinn (2004), Hispanic students prefer visual aids, as well as hands-on experience and inquiry. As indicated earlier, Hispanics are a collective culture and often prefer to work in groups. There is research to suggest the use of cohort groups is a useful strategy to ensure student success. Maldonado-Torres (2011) studied Dominican and Puerto Rican students in college and found that they preferred active experimentation and concrete experiences according to the Kolb Learning Style Inventory. The findings also suggest a preference for visual aids and tactile stimuli when learning, as well.

The use of learning technologies such as VC and simulation is thought to enhance student learning because these technologies are student-centered, involve collaborative learning, and engage students in the learning process. Early evidence shows that such approaches are especially appealing to minority students. This link may be explained by an emerging paradigm within higher education known as context diversity. According to Ibarra (2001), many elements within higher education environments are in conflict with the contexts of culturally diverse students. The theory of context diversity describes the need to create an academic learning community that not only attracts individuals from diverse cultures, but also allows them to thrive.

A concept of context diversity, multicontextuality, refers to a reframing of curricular and pedagogical practice by incorporating a variety of cognitive and cultural contexts (Ibarra, 2001). The concept of multicontextuality is based on cultural context and cognition research in which differences among cultures related to ways of seeing, interpreting, and communicating meaning from the world is reported (Hall, 1984). Many cultural groups, including Hispanics, rely on a multitude of communication cues (including verbal, nonverbal, interactions, and association) to understand the world around them — and thus are referred to as high context. The dominant cultural groups historically found in higher education (Anglo Americans) tend to rely on fewer communication modes (emphasizing words and analytical thinking) to understand the world around them — and thus are referred to as low context. These tendencies represent how individuals perceive, learn, and interact with the world around them. Many individuals demonstrate both low- and high-context preferences (or mixed) and are thus referred to as multicontextual. Approaches to teaching (lectures, reading), evaluation (written examinations, written papers), and assessment (standardized tests) in higher education have historically been consistent with the learning preferences of the low-context learner. Thus, academic performance may be more a reflection of performance as defined by the low-context perspective of higher education. Given this perspective, it is not difficult to understand why students with high-context preferences (as many Hispanic students are) face many challenges in nursing education. Giddens (2008) raises the idea that students who are labeled as "high-risk," may be so only in the current context of higher education.

Virtual communities and simulation are multi- and high-context learning applications; that is, they represent clinical situations involving people that require the application of knowledge to that situation. Students who have high-context preferences better understand nursing content that is nested in a situational clinical context. The theory of context diversity provides a framework for understanding the importance of incorporating a variety of learning approaches in the classroom to meet the learning needs of an increasingly diverse nursing student population.

### Strategies for Student Success

There are several key points integral to the success of Hispanic nursing students. All students appreciate being informed ahead of time of course expectations, which also applies to simulation. The pre-briefing is very important to Hispanic students because this allays many of the fears and or anxieties they may have going into simulation. English-as-a-second-language (ESL) students benefit greatly when given objectives and expected critical elements ahead of time. This allows the student an opportunity to look up words and definitions they may not be familiar with before entering the simulation. Avoiding the use of casual acronyms and abbreviations is also suggested because this may unnecessarily confuse the student.

Group dynamics are key in a successful simulation. Group assignments should be made based on grade point average and personal attributes, such as command of the English language and leadership skills. Role play and communication during the simulation are integral. Simulation may be one of the few opportunities the student has to make a "phone call" and inform the health care provider about their patient, without feeling embarrassed or worried about how he or she may sound to the other individual. If a student is embarrassed because of a heavy accent or perceived language barrier, having them interview the patient, deliver bad news, or educate the patient on a particular medication during the simulation provides students the opportunity to practice professional communication skills. By creating simulations that are contextually relevant to the didactic content or their own personal lives, the simulated experience takes on new meaning and becomes tangible to the high-context learner. Likewise, using simulated characters that are culturally similar to students brings home many of the key elements of the individual as a patient and provides familiarity, which enhances learning. For example, one Hispanic character in the Neighborhood, Mr. Reyes, has type one diabetes mellitus. When Mr. Reyes is used for the diabetic ketoacidosis simulation, a moment of immediate recognition occurs for some students; oftentimes Hispanic students will comment that Mr. Reyes has diabetes "like my grandfather" or "like my uncle." This reinforces the point that linking situations to context makes the learning experiences more relevant; thus, deeper learning occurs.

The post simulation debrief is crucial when working with Hispanic students; the ability to deconstruct the simulation and identify areas of self-improvement is vital to student success. Students may prefer to meet in private with the faculty member to review what the student may or may not have been comfortable with or understood. Even in the most supportive environment, the Hispanic student may appreciate an opportunity to debrief in private. Whenever possible the faculty member or simulation facilitator should try to accommodate this request.

## CONCLUSIONS AND RECOMMENDATIONS FOR NURSING EDUCATION

As the nation experiences an unprecedented growth in the Hispanic population, health care will need to meet the unique challenges of this ethnic group. Patient outcomes improve when a culturally competent health care provider or a "like-provider" is caring for them (Institute of Medicine, 2004; Sullivan Commission on Diversity in the Healthcare Workforce, 2004). One recommendation is to increase the number of Hispanic registered nurses. This will require ongoing efforts to increase the number of Hispanic students admitted to nursing programs. Schools of nursing have a responsibility to provide a learning environment and teaching strategies to facilitate the success of its Hispanic student nurse population. The use of innovative technologies, such as virtual communities and simulation, are just a couple of the strategies that can be useful in retaining and ensuring Hispanic nursing student success.

# REFERENCES

American Association of Colleges of Nurses. (2010). *Race/Ethnicity data on students enrolled in nursing programs* [Data file]. Retrieved from http://www.aacn.nche.edu/diversity-in-nursing

Benner, P., Sutphen, M., Leonard, V., & Day, L. (2010). *Educating nurses: A call for radical transformation.* San Francisco, CA: Jossey-Bass.

Carlson-Sabelli, J., Giddens, J., Fogg, L., & Fiedler, R. (2011). Challenges and benefits of using a virtual community to explore nursing concepts among baccalaureate nursing students. *International Journal of Nursing Education Scholarship, 8*(1), 1-14. doi:10.2202/1548-923X.2136

Curran, R., Elfrink, V., & Mays, B. (2009). Building a virtual community for nursing education: The town of Mirror Lake. *Journal of Nursing Education, 48*(1), 30-35.

Flinn, J. B. (2004). Teaching strategies used with success in the multicultural classroom. *Nurse Educator, 29*(1), 10-12.

Fogg, L., Carlson-Sabelli, L., Carlson, K., & Giddens, J. (in press). Perceived benefit of a virtual community based on learning styles, race-ethnicity, and frequency of use among nursing students. *Nursing Education Perspectives.*

Gates, M. G., Parr, M. B., & Hughen, J. (2012). Enhancing nursing knowledge Using high-fidelity simulation. *Journal of Nursing Education, 51*(1), 9-15.

Garrett, B., MacPhee, M., & Jackson, C. (2010). High-fidelity patient simulation: Considerations for effective learning. *Nursing Education Perspectives, 31*(5), 309-313.

Giddens, J. F. (2007). The Neighborhood. A web-based platform to support conceptual teaching and learning. *Nursing Education Perspectives, 28*(5), 251-256.

Giddens, J. F. (2008). Achieving diversity in nursing through multicontextual learning environments. *Nursing Outlook, 56*(2), 78-83.

Giddens, J., Fogg, L., & Carlson-Sabelli, L. (2010). Learning and engagement with a virtual community by undergraduate nursing students. *Nursing Outlook, 58*(5), 261-267.

Giddens, J., Hrabe, D., Carlson-Sabelli, L., Fogg, L., & North, S. (in press). The impact of a virtual community on student engagement and academic performance among baccalaureate nursing students. *Journal of Professional Nursing.*

Giddens, J., North, S., Carlson-Sabelli, L., Rogers, E., & Fogg, L. (2012). Using a virtual community to enhance cultural awareness among nursing students. *Journal of Transcultural Nursing, 23*(2), 198-204.

Giddens, J., Shuster, G., & Roerigh, N. (2010). Early student outcomes associated with a virtual community for learning. *Journal of Nursing Education, 49*(6), 355-358.

Gonzalez, L., & Fenske, C. L. (2012) Use of a virtual community to contextualize learning activities. *Journal of Nursing Education, 51*(1), 38-41.

Hall, E. T. (1984). The dance of life: The other dimension of time. New York, NY: Anchor.

Health Resources and Services Administration. (2000). *The registered nurse population: Findings from the National Sample Survey of Registered Nurses.* Retrieved from ERIC database. (ED471274)

Health Resources and Services Administration. (2010). *The registered nurse population: Findings from the 2008 National Sample Survey of Registered Nurses.* Washington, DC: Author.

Ibarra, R. (2001). *Beyond affirmative action: Reframing the context of higher education.* Madison, WI: University of Wisconsin Press.

Institute of Medicine (2004). *In the nation's compelling interest. Ensuring diversity in the health-care workforce.* Washington, DC: National Academies Press.

Ironside, P., & Jeffries, P. (2010) Using multiple-patient simulation experiences to foster clinical judgment. *Journal of Nursing Regulation, 1*(2), 38-41.

Jeffries, P. (Ed.). (2007). *Simulation in nursing education.* New York, NY: National League for Nursing.

Kantor, S. A. (2010). Pedagogical changes in nursing education: One instructor's experience. *Journal of Nursing Education, 49*(7), 414-417.

Maldonado-Torres, S. E. (2011). Differences in learning styles of Dominican and Puerto Rican students: We are Latinos from the Caribbean; our first language is Spanish, however; our learning preferences are different. *Journal of Hispanic Higher Education, 10*(3), 226-236.

Micari, M., & Drane, D. (2011). Intimidation in small learning groups: The roles of social comparison concern, comfort, and individual characteristics in student academic outcomes. *Active Learning in Higher Education, 12*(3), 175-187.

Moceri, J. T. (2010) Being Cabezona: Success strategies of Hispanic nursing students. *International Journal of Nursing Education Scholarship, 7*(1), 1-15. doi:10.2202/1548-923X.2036

Pappamihiel, N. E., & Moreno, M. (2011). Retaining Latino students: Culturally responsive instruction in colleges and universities. *Journal of Hispanic Higher Education, 10*(4), 331-344.

Rizzolo, M. A., Oermann, M. H., Jeffries, P., & Kardong-Edgren. (2011). NLN project to explore use of simulation for high stakes assessment. *Clinical Simulation in Nursing, 7*(6), e261-e262. doi:10.1016/j.ecns.2011.09.062

Shuster, G., Giddens, J., & Roerigh, N. (2011). Emotional connection and integration: Dominant themes among undergraduate nursing students using a virtual community. *Journal of Nursing Education, 50*(4), 222-5. doi:10.3928/01484834-20110131-02

Sullivan Commission on Diversity in the Healthcare Workforce. (2004). Missing persons: Minorities in the health professions: *A report of the Sullivan Commission on Diversity in the Healthcare Workforce*. Washington, DC: Author.

United States Census Bureau. (2010). *USA Quick Facts*. Retrieved from http://quickfacts.census.gov/qfd/states/00000.html

Velez-McEvoy, M. (2010). Faculty role in retaining Hispanic nursing students. *Creative Nursing, 16*(2), 80-83.

Walsh, M. (2011). Narrative pedagogy and simulation: Future directions for nursing education. *Nurse Education in Practice, 11*(3), 216-219.

Walsh, M., & Crumbie, A. (2011). Initial evaluation of Stillwell: A multimedia virtual community. *Nurse Education in Practice, 11*(2), 136-140.

# APPENDIX A

## AUTHOR PROFILES

# ANTONIA M. VILLARRUEL, PhD, RN, FAAN

Antonia M. Villarruel is professor, Nola J. Pender Collegiate Chair, and associate dean for research and global affairs at the University of Michigan School of Nursing. As a bilingual and bicultural nurse researcher, she has extensive research and practice experience with diverse Latino and Mexican populations and communities and health promotion and health disparities research and practice. She has been the principal and co-principal investigator of seven randomized clinical trials concerned with reducing sexual and other risk behaviors. As part of this program of research, she developed an efficacious program, entitled ¡Cuidate!, to reduce sexual risk behavior among Latino youth. This program is disseminated nationally by the Centers for Disease Control and Prevention as part of their Diffusion of Evidence Based Interventions program. In addition to her research, Dr. Villarruel has assumed leadership in many national and local organizations. She is the past president and a founding member of the National Coalition of Ethnic Minority Nursing Associations and past president of the National Association of Hispanic Nurses. She has served as a member of the HRSA/CDC HIV/STD Advisory Council and also as a charter member of the Secretary of the Department of Health and Human Services' Advisory Council on Minority Health and Health Disparities. She currently serves as a member of the Strategic Advisory Council of the AARP/RWJ Future of Nursing Campaign for Action. She has received numerous honors and awards, including membership in the Institute of Medicine and selection as a fellow in the American Academy of Nursing.

# SARA TORRES, PhD, RN, FAAN

Sara Torres is nationally known for her research on interpersonal violence; she conducted one of the first comparative studies in the nation of Hispanic women's attitudes toward domestic violence. She has received funds from the National Institutes of Health, published numerous articles, and presented at state, national, and international conferences on domestic violence research. She is editor of a book, Hispanic Health Care Educators Speak Out, and co-founding editor of Hispanic Health Care International, the official journal of the National Association of Hispanic Nurses. Dr. Torres has received numerous awards, including the Surgeon General's Exemplary Service Award. Dr. Torres is a fellow of the American Academy of Nursing and a member of Sigma Xi, the Scientific Research Society. She is involved in international activities and served as a consultant on mental health nursing to the Pan American Health Organization; she was the director, World Health Organization Collaborating Center on Mental Health Nursing at the University of Maryland School of Nursing. Dr. Torres has served at the national level on committees of numerous associations, including the American Nurses Association, the American Academy of Nursing, the National League for Nursing, the Food and Drug Administration Psychopharmacologic Drugs Advisory Committee, the U.S. Department of Justice, the U.S. Department of Health and Human Services Violence Against Women Advisory Council, and the Centers for Disease Control Advisory Committee on Injury Prevention and Control. Furthermore, Dr. Torres is a past president of the National Association of Hispanic Nurses and served a two-year term on the New Jersey Board of Nursing.

## STEPHANIE ACOSTA

Stephanie Acosta is a nursing student at the University of Texas Health Science Center in San Antonio (UTHSCSA). After completing her associate's degree at the community college level, she enrolled in the UTHSCSA School of Nursing Traditional Baccalaureate program. She has participated in the Juntos Podemos (Together We Can) mentorship and credits it with providing her with the support needed to successfully complete the program.

## CARMEN ALVAREZ, PhD, RN, NP-C, CNM

Carmen Alvarez completed her doctoral education in 2012 at the University of Michigan. Her research focused on sexual communication among young adult heterosexual Latinos She is also a family nurse practitioner and midwife and earned her master's in nursing science from Emory University. During her doctoral training, she practiced as a nurse practitioner in a medically underserved area of Detroit. This double life of clinical practice and research has worked to inform both her research endeavors and clinical practice. Her clinical and research experience both in the United States and abroad has inspired her pursuit of a career that will focus on research and policy development related to enhancing health care access for underserved populations. Consistent with this career trajectory Dr. Alvarez was awarded the Julio Bellber Fellowship at George Washington University.

## JEAN ASHWILL, MSN, RN

Jean Ashwill is assistant dean for undergraduate student services at the University of Texas at Arlington School of Nursing. She has over 45 years of experience in nursing, specializing in pediatrics. She has been involved in nursing education since 1982. Ms. Ashwill has taught pediatric nursing, directed two continuing nursing education programs and in her current role is responsible for recruitment, admissions, retention, and student scholarships. She has co-authored two nursing texts, one of which received the American Journal of Nursing Book of the Year award. Ms. Ashwill has been involved in several grants that have focused on the recruitment and retention of students from disadvantaged backgrounds. Her commitment to student success directs her current role as assistant dean.

## SUSAN BAXLEY, PhD, RN

Susan Baxley has practiced nursing for over 43 years, specializing in maternal-infant health. Her expertise in education and mentoring of patients, staff, and students led her to a research focus with Mexican-origin women becoming mothers. Dr. Baxley worked on several projects related to Hispanics and mentoring, including two research grants with a focus on the success of diverse students. As a faculty in the MSN program teaching research and theory in nursing, she mentors students in their understanding of the research process. She serves as co-director of the PhD in nursing mentoring program, where she provides guidance and special programs to both protégés and mentors that help the protégés to become nurse scientists. This interest has led her to a new research focus on the mentoring of PhD students and their needs.

## RAQUEL ALICIA BENAVIDES-TORRES, PhD, MCE, BSN

Raquel Alicia Benavides-Torres is professor and research coordinator of the School of Nursing and manages the nursing unit at the Health Research Center at Universidad Autónoma de Nuevo León in Monterrey, Nuevo León, Mexico. She received her PhD from the University of Texas at Austin. Her professional and research interest is to prevent HIV/AIDS in vulnerable populations. Dr. Benavides has been the principal investigator and co-investigator of several funded studies by the National Center of HIV Prevention, the Health Council and the Public Health System in Mexico. Dr. Benavides is president elect of the Tau Alpha Chapter of Sigma Theta Tau International. She has been recognized as a researcher by the National Research System and the National Center of Science and Technology in Mexico. She has publications in different peer reviewed journals, book chapters, and one book; she has participated in national and international conferences.

## MARY LOU BOND, PhD, RN, CNE, ANEF, FAAN

Mary Lou Bond is the Samuel T. Hughes Professor of Nursing at the University of Texas at Arlington (UTA) College of Nursing. Dr. Bond holds a BSN from Texas Christian University (TCU), an MN from the University of Pittsburgh, and a PhD from the University of Texas at Austin, as well as a certificate in nurse-midwifery from the University of Puerto Rico. She has spent over 40 years in various faculty and administrative positions at UTA, the University of Arkansas for Medical Sciences, and TCU. In 2011 she was honored as the Outstanding Alumna of the University of Pittsburgh School of Nursing. Dr. Bond practiced nurse-midwifery in central Mexico for four years and upon her return to the United States began programs for recruitment, retention, progression, and graduation of Hispanic students. She is co-founder and co-director of the Center for Hispanic Studies in Nursing and Health at UTA.

# EVELYN RUIZ CALVILLO, DNSc, RN

Evelyn Calvillo is professor emeritus at the School of Nursing at California State University, Los Angeles. She was co-chair of the Cultural Competency Advisory Group that developed the American Association of Colleges of Nursing (AACN) Master's and Doctoral Nursing Cultural Competencies and participated in the development of the AACN Baccalaureate Cultural Competencies. She is currently on the steering committee for the development of the Healthcare Disparities and Cultural Competency Consensus Standards by the National Quality Forum. She has served on numerous boards and committees for a variety of nursing projects. She has made numerous presentations on conducting culturally competent research. She has conducted research with Latino populations with a focus on traditional health beliefs, most recently a National Institute of Health funded project at the City of Hope. She has served as a consultant on culturally competent research as an investigator for the Center for Vulnerable Populations Research, University of California, Los Angeles School of Nursing.

# ADELITA G. CANTU, PhD, RN

Adelita G. Cantu is a native of San Antonio, Texas. She received her BSN from the University of the Incarnate Word; her MS with a focus on community health nursing from Texas Women's University and her PhD in clinical nursing research from the University of Texas Health Science Center in San Antonio (UTHSCSA). Dr. Cantu works is an assistant professor in the Family and Community Health Systems at the UTHSCSA School of Nursing. Dr. Cantu is course coordinator for the undergraduate population-focused health course. Her research commitments are focused on understanding factors that contribute to health disparities, especially among low-income Mexican Americans. Dr. Cantu is very active in community service, serving on numerous boards and advisory panels the goals of which include healthy living in San Antonio and surrounding communities. She has been a past coordinator for a student mentoring program promoting academic success of at-risk nursing students and a faculty advisor to pre-nursing students.

# CAROLYN L. CASON, PhD, RN

Carolyn L. Cason joined the University of Texas (UT) at Arlington in January, 1997, as professor and associate dean for research, College of Nursing. She has over 35 years of teaching experience in schools of nursing and has taught in undergraduate and graduate programs. Throughout her career she has worked to increase diversity in the health care workforce. She is co-founder of the Smart HospitalTM, a physical virtual hospital, which serves as a teaching and research and development facility. She created the Genomics Translational Research Laboratory within the College of Nursing and, in collaboration with colleagues in the College of Engineering, developed Smart Care (a center dedicated to developing technology to enhance independent living). In November, 2011 she became interim vice president for research at UT Arlington.

## CLAUDIA S. COGGIN, PhD, CHES

Claudia S. Coggin has both a master's of science and doctor of philosophy from Texas Woman's University in health education and is a certified health education specialist. Dr. Coggin recently retired as assistant professor in the department of behavioral and community health and director of the center for public health practice at the University of North Texas Health Sciences Center School of Public Health. Dr. Coggin taught classes in the master's in public health program and the doctorate in public health program and placed and supervised MPH students in their public health practice experience sites. Areas of community-based participatory research interest include women's health, public health workforce development, and leadership development. Her areas of teaching expertise are community health education promotion program planning, effective health communication, health literacy strategies in the community, and the development of health education materials. Dr. Coggin is currently a private health education consultant.

## LINDA DENKE, PhD, RN

Linda Denke is a full-time professor of nursing at Collin College, named by the National League for Nursing (NLN) as a Center of Excellence (2012-2015) in Nursing Education. She is known for her scholarly teaching, nursing research, mentoring, and curricular achievements in medical surgical and mental health nursing. During her career, she has had the privilege of designing and delivering health care to those affected by AIDS, the Navajo people, and uninsured minority women. Her service to vulnerable, diverse groups includes her roles on the National League for Nursing Diversity Task Force and the Board of Directors for the National Association of Mental Illness Collin County. Her consistent leadership has earned her recent roles as vice president of Faculty Council and as a fellow in the Academy of College Excellence Fellowship.

## MAITHE ENRIQUEZ, PhD, RN, ANP-BC

Maithe Enriquez is associate professor, University of Missouri, Sinclair School of Nursing and nurse practitioner, Truman Medical Center-Hospital Hill. In 2009, she was awarded the Local Heroes Award by Bank of America, and in 2010, she was voted Faculty of the Year by the University of Missouri-Kansas City School of Nursing student body. She has focused her research and clinical career on enhancing health outcomes for underserved low-income individuals of color living with or at-risk for HIV and violence. Her academic service has focused on enhancing the success of low-income students and first-generation college students. Dr. Enriquez has been a mentor for the National Coalition of Ethnic Minority Nurse Associations and is currently treasurer for both the Kansas City Chapter of the Association of Nurses in AIDS Care and her local chapter of the National Association of Hispanic Nurses, El Corazon de la Tierra.

## ANTONIO R. FLORES, PhD

Antonio R. Flores is president and chief executive officer of the Hispanic Association of Colleges and Universities (HACU). Dr. Flores received his PhD in higher education administration from the University of Michigan-Ann Arbor, his Master of Arts degree in counseling and personnel from Western Michigan University. He received his undergraduate degree in business administration from the Universidad de Guadalajara and was trained in elementary education at the Centro Normal Regional, both in Mexico. Dr. Flores has extensive experience in the areas of higher education, administration, and research. Prior to his post at HACU he served as director of programs and services for the Michigan Higher Education Assistance Authority and the Michigan Higher Education Student Loan Authority. During Dr. Flores' tenure at HACU the organization has tripled its membership and budget, expanded its programs, and worked on legislation affecting Hispanic Serving Institutions (HSIs).

## ESTHER C. GALLEGOS, PhD, RN, MBA, BSN

Esther C. Gallegos is professor at Universidad Autónoma de Nuevo León, Mexico. She received a baccalaureate in nursing from Universidad Nacional de Colombia, a master's in business administration from Universidad Autónoma de Nuevo León, and a doctor of philosophy in nursing from Wayne State University in Detroit, Michigan. She was the first in Mexico to receive a PhD in nursing. Dr. Gallegos has taught in undergraduate and graduate programs. At the graduate level, she led the building of the curriculum for the master's and doctoral programs. Both programs have been pioneers in nursing education in Mexico. Her research interest is self-care in chronic diseases, including risk factors prevention. In 1998, Dr. Gallegos received the Isabel Cendala y Gómez National Award in Nursing from the Health Department, Mexico. She is a member of the American Academy of Nursing and of the National System of Researchers in Mexico.

## JEAN GIDDENS, PhD, RN, FAAN

Jean Giddens is professor and executive dean at the College of Nursing, University of New Mexico in Albuquerque, New Mexico, and is a Robert Wood Johnson Executive Nurse Fellow, 2011 Cohort. Dr. Giddens earned a bachelor of science in nursing from the University of

Kansas, a master's of science in nursing from the University of Texas at El Paso, and a doctorate in education and human resource studies from Colorado State University. Dr. Giddens' teaching experience includes associate-, baccalaureate-, and graduate-degree programs in New Mexico, Texas, and Colorado. She is an expert in concept-based curriculum development and evaluation, as well as innovative strategies for teaching and learning. Dr. Giddens is the author of multiple journal articles, nursing textbooks, and electronic media, and serves as an education consultant to nursing programs throughout the country.

## PAT GLEASON-WYNN, PhD, RN, LCSW

Pat Gleason-Wynn has a PhD in social work and a BSN from the University of Texas at Arlington. She is a licensed clinical social worker and a registered nurse. Dr. Gleason-Wynn has worked with older adults in various settings for the past 32 years. She is a consultant and lecturer on gerontology. Her particular practice and research interests are mental health, palliative/end-of-life care, and social work practice in long-term care. She is the co-chair of the Health Council of the United Way of Tarrant County, and presides on the advisory board of the Area Agency on Aging of Tarrant County. Dr. Gleason-Wynn is the current past-president of the Texas Chapter of the National Association of Social Workers. In addition, she is a cardiac-telemetry nurse at Harris Methodist Fort Worth, Texas, and a hospice nurse for Odyssey Hospice in Fort Worth.

## LAURA GONZALEZ, PhD, RN, APRN, CNE

Laura González is assistant professor at the University of Central Florida. She has taught medical-surgical nursing, fundamentals, pathophysiology, community health and leadership, and management. She has extensive experience with virtual communities and incorporating the use of electronic health records into curricula. She has been in academia for over 10 years and has held positions as director of simulation and virtual learning. Her areas of interest include the use of simulation in nursing education and the transfer of knowledge to the clinical setting. She is the education chair for the International Nursing Association for Clinical Simulation and Learning and a current simulation leader with the National League for Nursing. Dr. Gonzalez was recently awarded a $1.3 million dollar Health Resources and Services Administration funded grant entitled "Integrated Technology into Nursing Education and Practice," which focused on faculty development in the areas of simulation, electronic health records, and telehealth.

## ROSA M. GONZALEZ-GUARDA, PhD, MPH, RN, CPH

Rosa M. Gonzalez-Guarda is assistant professor at the University of Miami School of Nursing and Health Studies. She holds degrees from Georgetown University (BSN), Johns Hopkins University (MSN/MPH), and the University of Miami (PhD). Her research focuses on the intersection of substance abuse, intimate partner violence, and risky sexual behaviors among Hispanics and the development of culturally tailored interventions to address these. Dr. Gonzalez-Guarda has received several honors and awards, including the appointment to an Institute of Medicine Committee on the Future of Nursing, a cornerstone of the Robert Wood Johnson Foundation (RWJF) initiative on the Future of Nursing. She was also recently selected to be a RWJF Nurse Faculty Scholar. Through this program she will develop and pilot test a teen dating violence prevention program for Hispanic youth.

## JENNIFER GRAY, PhD, RN

Jennifer Gray is associate dean and chair, department of MSN administration, education, and PhD programs at the College of Nursing at the University of Texas at Arlington. In her administrative role, she is responsible for implementing curricula to prepare nurse administrators, educators, and scientists to improve health outcomes for culturally diverse and vulnerable populations. As the George W. and Hazel M. Jay Professor, she is leading a team of nurses providing research and professional development workshops in Uganda each summer. In addition to her experiences in Uganda, her work in Cameroon as a nurse for mobile clinic and in Tanzania as a consultant to a rural hospital has made her passionate about health care in Africa.

## MICHAEL LOPEZ, BA

Michael Lopez is student loan specialist at Everest College Fort Worth South. Mr. Lopez has had a career in education for almost 20 years. He has worked in all levels from elementary through higher education, including academic and non-profit organizations. While working for the University of Texas in Arlington School of Nursing from 1994-1997, he worked on a Health Resources and Services Administration grant through a program called STARS for Nursing. The program targeted students at specific high schools and encouraged them to consider a career in nursing after graduation. In addition to recruitment, the project provided resources to retain nursing students in the program, leading to the graduation of students who will provide culturally competent care to diverse patient populations. The program offered scholarships, peer mentoring, and academic assistance. Also, students were introduced to role model mentors — nurses already working in the community who were ethnically or racially like their mentees.

## ROBERT J. LUCERO, PhD, RN

Robert Lucero is assistant professor of nursing at the Columbia University School of Nursing. Dr. Lucero is originally from Arizona, where he practiced nursing among underserved, vulnerable Mexican families. He studied at the University of Pennsylvania and received a

PhD for his research on the patterns of nursing care and adverse events among hospitalized patients. Dr. Lucero is developing, implementing, and studying the use of health information technology (HIT) among predominately Latino populations in New York City. This research focuses on Latinos as consumers in the development of HIT for self-management. Dr. Lucero continues to conduct hospital-based research focused on identifying effective prevention interventions through the novel use of electronic clinical data. He is an affiliated member of the Center for Evidence-based Practice in the Underserved, the Center for Health Policy, and the Northern Manhattan Center of Excellence in Minority Health and Health Disparities at Columbia University.

## NORMA MARTINEZ ROGERS, PhD, RN, FAAN

A former resident of public housing, Norma Martinez Rogers has spent her life in service to the community as a nurse, educator, and an advocate for the underserved population. She obtained a master's of science in nursing and a PhD from the University of Texas in Austin in cultural foundations of education — a life-long dream of hers. Dr. Rogers started a mentorship program titled Juntos Podemos (Together We Can). This program began with 20 students and has grown to have 300 students, 98 percent of whom are academically successful; in the past six years, 100 percent of them passed NCLEX on their first attempt. Juntos Podemos has established undergraduate electives with a focus on being a research, teaching, or leadership scholar. The program has its own web domain at the University of Texas Health Sciences Center in San Antonio and this semester will have its own website entitled "For Future Nurses.com."

## EVE MCGEE, MSW

Eve McGee is a research associate at the University of Missouri-Kansas City School of Nursing, where she oversees a retention program for students who are underrepresented in health care professions. As director of social services for reStart Inc., one of the largest homeless shelters in the area, Ms. McGee was responsible for daily operations of the shelter and identifying community resources for clients. Ms. McGee has coordinated community-based projects including education, support, and mentoring for at-risk individuals and groups, such as the homeless, women living with HIV/AIDS, and families living in poverty. She currently serves on the REACH Healthcare Foundation Board of Directors and is the vice president of the Missouri-Kansas National Association of Black Social Workers. Ms. McGee has lectured on effective support for ethnically diverse students and how to increase cultural competency in nursing education.

# MICHAEL D. MOON, MSN, RN, CNS-CC, CEN, FAEN

Michael D. Moon is currently an instructor at the University of the Incarnate Word Ila Faye Miller School of Nursing where he teaches critical care nursing. In addition to his clinical nurse specialist role, Mr. Moon has held positions in academia, clinical practice, and management. Mr. Moon is currently completing his PhD. His dissertation focuses on new emergency nurses in practice. His research interests include underrepresented populations in nursing, nursing education, clinical instruction design, and emergency nursing practice. Mr. Moon currently serves on the Emergency Nurses Association Board of Directors. He holds a BSN from Texas Tech University Health Sciences Center and a MSN from the University of Texas Health Science Center at San Antonio. In addition, Mr. Moon is a certified emergency nurse and a fellow in the Academy of Emergency Nursing.

# LUSINE POGHOSYAN, PhD, RN

Lusine Poghosyan is assistant professor at Columbia University School of Nursing. Her research focuses on investigating nursing workforce issues in the U.S. and internationally. Her recent studies focus on investigating the nurse practitioner (NP) workforce in primary care settings and the impact of organizational climates on the NP workforce. Dr. Poghosyan developed a new research tool to measure organizational climate in primary care settings from the perspectives of nurse practitioners. Her international work focuses on investigating nursing practice in hospitals and finding ways to promote nursing practice, especially in post-Soviet countries. Her recent study investigated nursing practice in the hospitals of Armenia. Dr. Poghosyan completed her doctoral and post-doctoral training at the University of Pennsylvania, School of Nursing.

# BERTHA CECILIA SALAZAR-GONZÁLEZ, PhD, RN, MA, BSN

Bertha Cecilia Salazar-González has been a full-time professor at the School of Nursing, Universidad Autónoma de Nuevo León (UANL) since 1979. Her administrative position as doctoral program coordinator started in 2010; from 2000-2009 she was responsible for the research office. She serves as president for Tau-Alpha Chapter (STTI) 2010-2012. She received a baccalaureate in nursing from Universidad de Monterrey, a master's in higher education from Universidad Regiomontana, and a doctor of philosophy from Wayne State University. Dr. Salazar-González belongs to the National Researcher System: Level II 2008-2012 and serves on demand as peer review for national and UANL research proposals applying for grants. Her research interest is in physical and cognitive function in older adults. She is currently conducting an intervention aimed to improved elders' abilities to walk concurrently to a cognitive task. Dr. Salazar-González has served as chair for 20 master's students and seven doctoral students.

## ELIZABETH TREVINO DAWSON, DrPH, MPH

Dr. Elizabeth Trevino Dawson obtained her DrPH in health management and policy from the University of North Texas Health Science Center (UNTHSC). She is assistant dean for curriculum, director for the master's of health administration program, and assistant professor at UNTHSC School of Public Health. As part of her role, she is advisor and mentor to over 30 aspiring health care leaders in the master of health administration program. Dr. Trevino's interests focus on health disparities, health care status, and utilization of health care services for vulnerable populations. Dr. Trevino is a collaborator in the implementation of a Diabetes Disease Management program whose goal is to improve access to quality diabetes care and health outcomes for the uninsured and underserved in Tarrant County. Dr. Trevino was recipient of the Fort Worth Business Press Award "40 under 40" which honors individuals shaping the future of Tarrant County through business and community involvement.

## THERESA VILLARREAL, MSN, RN, ACNS-BC

Theresa Villarreal is clinical assistant professor at the University of Texas Health Science Center at San Antonio. She is also faculty advisor for Juntos Podemos (Together We Can) and Juntos Avanzamos (Together We Advance). As faculty adviser, she assists pre-nursing and nursing students to succeed in their progression through the academic program. As clinical assistant professor, she manages nursing students in clinical rotations, including on unit observation, clinical skills lab, and classroom teaching. She also coordinates with clinical site personnel to create an enhanced student learning experience. Ms. Villarreal has been a nurse for 14 years and a nurse educator more than five years.

# APPENDIX B

## INSTRUCTIONAL SELF-ASSESSMENT

## University of Texas Arlington Institutional Self-Assessment for Factors Supporting Hispanic Student Recruitment and Persistence

*In Cason, C. L., Bond, M. L., & Gleason-Wynn, P. (2007). Institutional self-assessment for factors supporting Hispanic student recruitment and persistence. Arlington, TX: School of Nursing, University of Texas at Arlington. Permission to reprint from Cason, Bond & Gleason-Wynn.*

### Scoring Instructions:

For each item within each section select the descriptor that is most like your program. The value associated with that descriptor is noted at the top of the column in which the descriptor appears. A summed score on the assessment ranges from 25 to 100. Higher scores suggest that the program holds the characteristics of a program that supports Hispanic student recruitment and persistence. Calculating an average score for each construct may be helpful in developing a plan for promoting student success, as the scores provide a profile of program strengths and opportunities for improvement. The table provided here can be used to record total scores for each construct and calculate the average.

| Construct | Total Score on Items for that Construct | Divide by # of Items | Construct Score |
|---|---|---|---|
| Financial Support and Opportunity | | 4 | |
| Emotional and Moral Support | | 7 | |
| Mentoring | | 3 | |
| Academic Advising | | 3 | |
| Technical Support | | 4 | |
| Professional Socialization | | 4 | |

| | Low | | | High |
|---|---|---|---|---|
| | **Financial Support and Opportunity** | | | |
| | 1 | 2 | 3 | 4 |
| Item 1 | Students must seek information about financial support that is available. | Students are provided information about financial support that is available. | Students are encouraged to apply for financial support that is available (if requested, assistance is provided in completing forms and obtaining information). | Students are provided information about funding that is available, matched to sources of funding, and assisted in making application (assistance in completing forms and obtaining information is offered). |
| Item 2 | No scholarships or stipends are available through the school for minority students. | Limited scholarships or stipends are available through the school for minority students. | Some scholarships or stipends are available through the school for minority students. | Number of students receiving scholarships is parallel to percentage of minority students. |
| Item 3 | Criteria for receiving scholarship or stipend are unrelated to minority students or GPA. | Primary criterion for receiving scholarship or stipend is GPA. | Criteria include financial need or non-grade related achievements. | Criteria include consideration of minority status, GPA, and non-grade related achievements. |
| Item 4 | Financial support is limited to payment of tuition and fees. | Financial support includes scholarships and stipends that can pay for tuition, fees, and other school-related expenses including housing and living expenses. | Financial support includes scholarships, stipends, and cooperative work opportunities designed to accommodate student's schedule. | Financial support includes a broad range of funding sources such as scholarships, stipends, cooperative programs with industrial/business partners, and loan forgiveness programs to minimize the number of hours a student must work each week. |

| | Low | | | High |
|---|---|---|---|---|
| | **Emotional and Moral Support** | | | |
| | 1 | 2 | 3 | 4 |
| Item 1 | Faculty and staff are abrupt and cool during interactions with students. | Staff and faculty are professional but distant in their interactions with students. | Staff and faculty are pleasant and friendly with students and families but are task-focused during interactions. | Staff and faculty create a welcoming environment by being genuinely interested in students and their families. |
| Item 2 | Faculty members are unavailable to students outside the classroom. | Faculty members are available only during office hours to meet with students and to talk to them by telephone. | Faculty members are available by appointment to meet with students and to talk by telephone. | Faculty members encourage students to meet with them and have an open door policy. |
| Item 3 | Faculty members are abrupt and distant with students in classroom and clinical environments. | Faculty members are polite and professional with students in classroom and clinical environments. | Faculty members convey their interest in students' professional growth during interactions in classroom and clinical environments. | Faculty members convey their interest in students as people and future colleagues during interactions in classroom and clinical environments. |
| Item 4 | Faculty and staff observe that students make unsupportive or discriminatory comments in their interactions with peers. | Faculty and staff observe that students are neutral and passive in their interactions with their peers, rarely interacting with each other outside of classes or required project activities. | Faculty and staff observe that a few students interact with each other outside of classes or required project activities and provide limited emotional support. | Faculty and staff observe that most students support each other outside of classes and in required project activities. |

| | Low | | | High |
|---|---|---|---|---|
| | **Emotional and Moral Support** | | | |
| | 1 | 2 | 3 | 4 |
| Item 5 | Faculty and staff make no attempts to assess their own commitment to provide emotional and moral support. | Faculty and staff recognize students' need for faculty, peer, and family support for successful completion. | Faculty and staff assess the specific needs of students for emotional and moral support. | Faculty and staff build programs of institutional support which respond to the assessed needs. |
| Item 6 | Faculty and staff lack insight into cultural values of others. | Faculty and staff are aware of cultural values of underrepresented minorities | Faculty and staff provide culturally-appropriate communication with students. | Faculty and staff design activities and courses inclusive and supportive of cultural values and provide opportunity for ethnic expression and exploration. |
| Item 7 | Faculty and staff view students' families and friends as barriers to school success. | Faculty and staff view students' families and friends as neutral factors in school success. | Faculty and staff acknowledge students' families and friends as partners and they are invited to participate in social activities provided by the school. | Faculty and staff acknowledge students' families and friends as partners and they are encouraged to participate in school orientation and annual program updates. |

| | Low | | | High |
|---|---|---|---|---|
| | **Mentoring** | | | |
| | 1 | 2 | 3 | 4 |
| Item 1 | Administrators do not mention mentoring activities in program reports. | Administrators mention mentoring activities in program reports. | Administrators describe mentoring activities as the number of matches and number of contacts between mentors/mentees. | Administrators describe mentoring activities by satisfaction and outcomes of mentees and mentors. |
| Item 2 | Students are not assigned mentors within the academic program. | Students are assigned mentors within the academic program. | Students are matched to a mentor based on race/ ethnicity and area of expertise. | Students are matched to a mentor based on race/ ethnicity and area of expertise. Students and mentors evaluate the match for fit. Students may self-select mentors. |
| Item 3 | Mentors are expected to know about mentoring from their own life and academic experiences. | Mentors are provided mentoring guidelines. | Mentors are provided an initial orientation to role of mentor. | Mentors are provided an initial orientation and periodic refresher learning opportunities based on mentor and mentee feedback. |

| Low | | | High |
|-----|-----|-----|-----|
| **Academic Advising** | | | |
| 1 | 2 | 3 | 4 |
| **Item 1** A student may request academic advising and see the advisor that is available at that time. | Each student is required to meet with an academic advisor once a semester. | Each student is linked to an academic advisor when he or she is admitted to the educational program and continues to see that advisor each semester unless the student requests a change. | Each student is linked to an academic advisor during the recruitment phase and continues to see that advisor through graduation unless the student requests a change. |
| **Item 2** Academic advising services are not available. | Academic advisors approve the initial degree plan and any changes. | Academic advisors give students permission to enroll in courses each semester and use a prescriptive approach to advising. | Academic advisors provide course, program, and career guidance using a developmental approach to advising. |
| **Item 3** Academic advisors are limited to a single ethnic group and/ or uninformed about needs of a diverse student population | Academic advisors acknowledge need for orientation to the needs of a diverse student population | Academic advisors recruited from a range of backgrounds; initial/ ongoing development programs related to needs of diverse student populations provided. | Pool of advisors includes persons from a range of backgrounds representative of student population and knowledgeable about cultural values and needs. |

| Low | | | High |
|-----|-----|-----|------|
| **Technical Support** | | | |
| 1 | 2 | 3 | 4 |
| **Item 1** Few computers are available for student use or, if adequate number, are available only during business hours. | Computers are available for student use in one or two locations on campus. | Computers are available for student use in most buildings on campus. | Computers are available for student use 24 hours daily in at least one location on campus. |
| **Item 2** Assistance with computer problems is not available to students. | Assistance with computer problems is available to students during office hours. | Assistance with computer problems is available to students during day/evening weekdays. | Assistance with computer problems is available to students 24 hours daily. |
| **Item 3** Computer accessibility is limited to computers available on campus. | Computer accessibility includes computers on campus for use or purchase at market cost. | Computer access for students is facilitated by options to rent a laptop or buy one at a reduced cost. | A laptop is provided to all students at admission with cost included in tuition and fees. |
| **Item 4** Student computer competency is not evaluated. | Student computer competency is evaluated. Students are made aware of available remedial courses to improve skills. | Student computer competency is evaluated. Students required or strongly encouraged to participate in standard workshops/courses to improve skills. | Student computer competency is evaluated. Workshops/courses are provided within the program to address identified student needs. |

| Low | | | High |
|-----|---|---|------|
| **Professional Socialization** | | | |
| 1 | 2 | 3 | 4 |
| **Item 1** Cultural values are negated if not congruent with professional values. Professional values take precedence over cultural values. | Cultural values are acknowledged but professional values are promoted. | Cultural values and professional values are encouraged equally, but remain distinct. | Professional values integrate and support cultural values. |
| **Item 2** Activities to promote professional socialization are not part of the curriculum. | Activities to promote professional socialization are course requirements in selected courses. | Activities to promote professional socialization are encouraged across the curriculum. | Activities to promote professional socialization are integrated throughout the curriculum and in community and campus activities. |
| **Item 3** Faculty are not involved in professional organizations. | Faculty are members of professional organizations and encourage student attendance at events. | Faculty are leaders in professional organizations and encourage student involvement. | Faculty are leaders in professional organizations and involve students in planning and implementing the activities. |
| **Item 4** Administrators and faculty do not recognize need for role models who are persons from underrepresented minorities. | Administrators and faculty recognize need for role models from persons who are underrepresented minorities. | Administrators and faculty actively recruit persons to serve as role models and resource persons to students. | Administrators and faculty facilitate student access to available and accessible professional role models, some of whom are persons from underrepresented minorities. |

*Funded by the National League for Nursing (Nursing Research Education Grant) and Texas Organization of Baccalaureate and Graduate Nursing Education (Excellence in Research Award)*

# APPENDIX C

## PROGRAM SELF-ASSESSMENT

## UNIVERSITY OF TEXAS ARLINGTON HEALTHCARE PROFESSIONS EDUCATION PROGRAM SELF-ASSESSMENT

*In Gray, J. R., Bond, M. L., & Cason, C. L. (2007b). Healthcare profession education program self-assessment (revised). Arlington, TX: College of Nursing, University of Texas at Arlington. Permission to reprint from Gray, Bond, & Cason.*

### Scoring Instructions:

For each item within each section select the descriptor that is most like your program. The value associated with that descriptor is noted at the top of the column in which the descriptor appears. A summed score on the assessment ranges from 25 to 100. Higher scores suggest that the program holds the characteristics of a program that supports Hispanic student recruitment and persistence. Calculating an average score for each construct may be helpful in developing a plan for promoting student success, as the scores provide a profile of program strengths and opportunities for improvement. The table provided here can be used to record total scores for each construct and calculate the average.

| Construct | Total Score on Items for that Construct | Divide by # of Items | Construct Score |
|---|---|---|---|
| Financial Support and Opportunity | | 4 | |
| Emotional and Moral Support | | 7 | |
| Mentoring | | 3 | |
| Academic Advising | | 3 | |
| Technical Support | | 4 | |
| Professional Socialization | | 4 | |

| | Low | | | High |
|---|---|---|---|---|
| | **Financial Support and Opportunity** | | | |
| | 1 | 2 | 3 | 4 |
| Item 1 | Students must seek information about financial support that is available. | Students are provided information about financial support that is available. | Students are encouraged to apply for financial support that is available (if requested, assistance is provided in completing forms and obtaining information). | Students are provided information about funding that is available, matched to sources of funding, and assisted in making application (assistance in completing forms and obtaining information is offered). |
| Item 2 | No scholarships or stipends are available through the school for minority students. | Limited scholarships or stipends are available through the school for minority students. | Some scholarships or stipends are available through the school for minority students. | Number of students receiving scholarships is parallel to percentage of minority students. |
| Item 3 | Criteria for receiving scholarship or stipend are unrelated to minority students or GPA. | Primary criterion for receiving scholarship or stipend is GPA. | Criteria include financial need or non-grade related achievements. | Criteria include consideration of minority status, GPA, and non-grade related achievements. |
| Item 4 | Financial support is limited to payment of tuition and fees. | Financial support includes scholarships and stipends that can pay for tuition, fees, and other school-related expenses including housing and living expenses. | Financial support includes scholarships, stipends, and cooperative work opportunities designed to accommodate student's schedule. | Financial support includes a broad range of funding sources such as scholarships, stipends, cooperative programs with industrial/business partners, and loan forgiveness programs to minimize the number of hours a student must work each week. |

| Low | | | High |
|---|---|---|---|
| **Emotional and Moral Support** | | | |
| 1 | 2 | 3 | 4 |
| **Item 1** Faculty and staff are abrupt and cool during interactions with students. | Staff and faculty are professional but distant in their interactions with students. | Staff and faculty are pleasant and friendly with students and families but are task-focused during interactions. | Staff and faculty create a welcoming environment by being genuinely interested in students and their families. |
| **Item 2** Faculty members are unavailable to students outside the classroom. | Faculty members are available only during office hours to meet with students and to talk to them by telephone. | Faculty members are available by appointment to meet with students and to talk by telephone. | Faculty members encourage students to meet with them and have an open door policy. |
| **Item 3** Faculty members are abrupt and distant with students in classroom and clinical environments. | Faculty members are polite and professional with students in classroom and clinical environments. | Faculty members convey their interest in students' professional growth during interactions in classroom and clinical environments. | Faculty members convey their interest in students as people and future colleagues during interactions in classroom and clinical environments. |
| **Item 4** Faculty and staff observe that students make unsupportive or discriminatory comments in their interactions with peers. | Faculty and staff observe that students are neutral and passive in their interactions with their peers, rarely interacting with each other outside of classes or required project activities. | Faculty and staff observe that a few students interact with each other outside of classes or required project activities and provide limited emotional support. | Faculty and staff observe that most students support each other outside of classes and in required project activities. |

| | Low | | | High |
|---|---|---|---|---|
| | **Emotional and Moral Support** | | | |
| | 1 | 2 | 3 | 4 |
| Item 5 | Faculty and staff make no attempts to assess their own commitment to provide emotional and moral support. | Faculty and staff recognize students' need for faculty, peer, and family support for successful completion. | Faculty and staff assess the specific needs of students for emotional and moral support. | Faculty and staff build programs of institutional support which respond to the assessed needs. |
| Item 6 | Faculty and staff lack insight into cultural values of others. | Faculty and staff are aware of cultural values of underrepresented minorities | Faculty and staff provide culturally-appropriate communication with students. | Faculty and staff design activities and courses inclusive and supportive of cultural values and provide opportunity for ethnic expression and exploration. |
| Item 7 | Faculty and staff view students' families and friends as barriers to school success. | Faculty and staff view students' families and friends as neutral factors in school success. | Faculty and staff acknowledge students' families and friends as partners and they are invited to participate in social activities provided by the school. | Faculty and staff acknowledge students' families and friends as partners and they are encouraged to participate in school orientation and annual program updates. |

| Low | | | High |
|-----|-----|-----|-----|
| **Mentoring** | | | |
| 1 | 2 | 3 | 4 |
| **Item 1** Administrators do not mention mentoring activities in program reports. | Administrators mention mentoring activities in program reports. | Administrators describe mentoring activities as the number of matches and number of contacts between mentors/mentees. | Administrators describe mentoring activities by satisfaction and outcomes of mentees and mentors. |
| **Item 2** Students are not assigned mentors within the academic program. | Students are assigned mentors within the academic program. | Students are matched to a mentor based on race/ ethnicity and area of expertise. | Students are matched to a mentor based on race/ ethnicity and area of expertise. Students and mentors evaluate the match for fit. Students may self-select mentors. |
| **Item 3** Mentors are expected to know about mentoring from their own life and academic experiences. | Mentors are provided mentoring guidelines. | Mentors are provided an initial orientation to role of mentor. | Mentors are provided an initial orientation and periodic refresher learning opportunities based on mentor and mentee feedback. |

| Low | | | High |
|-----|-----|-----|-----|
| **Academic Advising** | | | |
| 1 | 2 | 3 | 4 |
| **Item 1** A student may request academic advising and see the advisor that is available at that time. | Each student is required to meet with an academic advisor once a semester. | Each student is linked to an academic advisor when he or she is admitted to the educational program and continues to see that advisor each semester unless the student requests a change. | Each student is linked to an academic advisor during the recruitment phase and continues to see that advisor through graduation unless the student requests a change. |
| **Item 2** Academic advising services are not available. | Academic advisors approve the initial degree plan and any changes. | Academic advisors give students permission to enroll in courses each semester and use a prescriptive approach to advising. | Academic advisors provide course, program, and career guidance using a developmental approach to advising. |
| **Item 3** Academic advisors are limited to a single ethnic group and/ or uninformed about needs of a diverse student population | Academic advisors acknowledge need for orientation to the needs of a diverse student population | Academic advisors recruited from a range of backgrounds; initial/ ongoing development programs related to needs of diverse student populations provided. | Pool of advisors includes persons from a range of backgrounds representative of student population and knowledgeable about cultural values and needs. |

| | Low | | | High |
|---|---|---|---|---|
| | **Technical Support** | | | |
| | 1 | 2 | 3 | 4 |
| Item 1 | Few computers are available for student use or, if adequate number, are available only during business hours. | Computers are available for student use in one or two locations on campus. | Computers are available for student use in most buildings on campus. | Computers are available for student use 24 hours daily in at least one location on campus. |
| Item 2 | Assistance with computer problems is not available to students. | Assistance with computer problems is available to students during office hours. | Assistance with computer problems is available to students during day/evening weekdays. | Assistance with computer problems is available to students 24 hours daily. |
| Item 3 | Computer accessibility is limited to computers available on campus. | Computer accessibility includes computers on campus for use or purchase at market cost. | Computer access for students is facilitated by options to rent a laptop or buy one at a reduced cost. | A laptop is provided to all students at admission with cost included in tuition and fees. |
| Item 4 | Student computer competency is not evaluated. | Student computer competency is evaluated. Students are made aware of available remedial courses to improve skills. | Student computer competency is evaluated. Students required or strongly encouraged to participate in standard workshops/courses to improve skills. | Student computer competency is evaluated. Workshops/courses are provided within the program to address identified student needs. |

| | Low | | | High |
|---|---|---|---|---|
| | **Professional Socialization** | | | |
| | 1 | 2 | 3 | 4 |
| Item 1 | Cultural values are negated if not congruent with professional values. Professional values take precedence over cultural values. | Cultural values are acknowledged but professional values are promoted. | Cultural values and professional values are encouraged equally, but remain distinct. | Professional values integrate and support cultural values. |
| Item 2 | Activities to promote professional socialization are not part of the curriculum. | Activities to promote professional socialization are course requirements in selected courses. | Activities to promote professional socialization are encouraged across the curriculum. | Activities to promote professional socialization are integrated throughout the curriculum and in community and campus activities. |
| Item 3 | Faculty are not involved in professional organizations. | Faculty are members of professional organizations and encourage student attendance at events. | Faculty are leaders in professional organizations and encourage student involvement. | Faculty are leaders in professional organizations and involve students in planning and implementing the activities. |
| Item 4 | Administrators and faculty do not recognize need for role models who are persons from underrepresented minorities. | Administrators and faculty recognize need for role models from persons who are underrepresented minorities. | Administrators and faculty actively recruit persons to serve as role models and resource persons to students. | Administrators and faculty facilitate student access to available and accessible professional role models, some of whom are persons from underrepresented minorities. |

*Funded by the National League for Nursing (Nursing Research Education Grant) and Texas Organization of Baccalaureate and Graduate Nursing Education (Excellence in Research Award)*